Public Health Papers

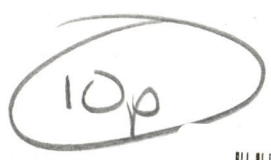

No. 76

The risk approach in health care

With special reference to maternal and child health, including family planning

Nurse Education Centre
City General Hospital
Newcastle Road
Stoke-on-Trent, ST4 6QG

The risk approach in health care

With special reference to maternal and child health, including family planning

E. Maurice Backett
Professor Emeritus, Department of Community Health,
The University of Nottingham Medical School,
Nottingham, England

A. Michael Davies
Professor of Medical Ecology,
Hadassah School of Public Health,
The Hebrew University, Jerusalem, Israel

Angèle Petros-Barvazian
Director, Division of Family Health,
World Health Organization,
Geneva, Switzerland

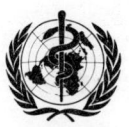

WORLD HEALTH ORGANIZATION
GENEVA
1984

ISBN 92 4 130076 0

© World Health Organization 1984

Publication of the World Health Organization enjoy copyright protection in accordance with the provisions of Protocol 2 of the Universal Copyright Convention. For rights of reproduction or translation of WHO publications, in part or *in toto*, application should be made to the Office of Publications, World Health Organization, Geneva, Switzerland. The World Health Organization welcomes such applications.

The designations employed and the presentation of the material in this publication do not imply the expression of any opinion whatsoever on the part of the Secretariat of the World Health Organization concerning the legal status of any country, territory, city or area or of its authorities, or concerning the delimitation of its frontiers or boundaries.

The mention of specific companies or of certain manufacturers' products does not imply that they are endorsed or recommended by the World Health Organization in preference to others of a similar nature that are not mentioned. Errors and omissions excepted, the names of proprietary products are distinguished by initial capital letters.

The authors alone are responsible for the views expressed in this publication.

TYPESET IN INDIA
PRINTED IN ENGLAND
83/5728 – Macmillan/Clays – 8000

Contents

	Page
Foreword	vii

1. INTRODUCTION ... 1
   1.1 Risk as a proxy for need ... 1
   1.2 Preventive medicine becomes more numerate ... 2
   1.3 The risk approach and the contribution of health services ... 4
   1.4 Predicting health ... 5

2. PROMOTING THE HEALTH OF MOTHERS AND CHILDREN ... 7
   2.1 The risk approach applied to maternal and child health ... 7
   2.2 Health problems and the concepts of risk and chance ... 8
   2.3 The potential of the risk approach ... 15

3. OUTCOME, RISK AND MEASUREMENT ... 18
   3.1 The data base ... 18
   3.2 Priorities among outcomes ... 19
   3.3 The measurement of risk ... 20
   3.4 Identifying the risk factors and the populations and individuals at risk ... 23
   3.5 "False positives" and "false negatives" and cost-benefit questions ... 29

4. FROM RISK MEASUREMENT TO INTERVENTION ... 32
   4.1 Preparatory steps ... 32
   4.2 The health care system: How can it be changed? ... 38
   4.3 Intervention at different levels of care ... 41

5. USES OF THE RISK APPROACH ... 43
   5.1 Applying the risk idea ... 43

5.2	Applications outside the organized system of care	44
5.3	Applications within the organized system of care	47
6.	**SELECTING INTERVENTIONS**	60
6.1	The potential for change in health care	60
6.2	Criteria for selection	61
6.3	Local priorities for action	62
6.4	Local resources	62
6.5	National priorities for action	63
6.6	A decision pathway	64
7.	**MONITORING AND EVALUATION**	68
7.1	Introduction	68
7.2	Monitoring health and health care	69
7.3	Appropriate health systems research and the obligation to inquire	70
7.4	Steps in a study protocol	71
7.5	Evaluation as part of health systems research	72
7.6	Routine evaluation of a service innovation	73
7.7	Evaluation criteria	74
8.	**LESSONS FROM THE RISK APPROACH**	79
8.1	Application to the whole field of primary health care	79
8.2	Impediments and barriers	81
8.3	Redressing inequalities in health: a strategy for improving primary health care	83

References 85

Acknowledgements 87

Annex 1. Selecting target health problems 91

Annex 2. A note on risk measurements 93

Annex 3. Annotated bibliography 104

Summary 111

Foreword

This book is more speculative than its predecessor, *Risk approach for maternal and child health care*,[1] of which it is to some extent a follow-up. It presents eight suggestions for the use of risk information in health care. Most of these still have to be tested in the real world with populations from village communities, migrants, nomads, and the inhabitants of urban slums, where mothers and children are at their most vulnerable and health systems research is the most difficult. These ideas come from a realization that in the accurate measurement of the chances of the occurrence of a future event, of health, or of illness, primary health care has a new tool with which to improve its effectiveness, its efficiency and its decisions about national and local priorities. The risk approach therefore lies at the very heart of primary health care; its potential is great but it remains to be seen how well it can be applied.

We start with the idea that a measure of risk is a proxy for need—need for promotive and preventive care—and the fact that knowledge available before the predicted event allows time for a proportionate response; hence we coin the slogan: "Something for all, but more for those in need—*in proportion to that need*".

This approach aims to redress the inequalities in health that afflict almost all societies, and is pragmatic in that it seeks social justice in health. Human and other resources should go where the need is greatest, and assessment of the risk of future illness, accident or death is a useful short cut to the measurement of that need—both for individuals and for communities. The risk approach should serve to concentrate care on the family itself, as well as to ensure that individuals are referred to the correct person or institution in the care system. It should also provide guidelines for training, and, by furnishing a community profile, act as a rough-and-ready guide to social policies for health.

Risk data come in different guises, the familiar *relative risk* and the more esoteric *attributable risk* being the best known. Of these two, the first is well suited for use at the individual level in helping us to

---

[1] WHO Offset Publication No. 39, Geneva, World Health Organization, 1978.

understand and react to danger signals, to refer ourselves for help when necessary, or to guide resource use to the optimum. The second type of risk information, however, is probably the most challenging, since this concept of *attribution* (though it must be approached with statistical and other reservations) provides a measure of what *could* happen to the community's health if the risk factors were removed. An instrument of health and social policy with this potential, even if it still remains to be developed and simplified, must be respected and its use is mandatory.

Because of the need for sophisticated epidemiology and statistics in testing the usefulness of the new risk information, general and technical training programmes are being developed on health systems research and the use of risk data in general. This book is intended as an introduction to both types of programme and is thus directed at specialists as well as generalists. In particular, it presents a series of hypotheses which, it is hoped, will stimulate all health workers who are facing the challenge of "health for all"—true development of health care systems.

Maurice Backett
Michael Davies
Angèle Petros-Barvazian

1. Introduction

1.1 Risk as a Proxy for Need

In every society there are communities, families and individuals whose chances of future illness, accident and untimely death are greater than those of others; these are said to be especially vulnerable and the reasons for this, though often tenuous, can usually be traced. There are also communities, families and individuals whose chance of being healthier than others is greater. Because most people are concerned more with the threat of illness than with health, the notion of risk has become part of our thinking about the prevention of disease—the chances of health being thought of mainly as a low risk of illness. We do not speak of our "vulnerability to health" and epidemiologists rarely study the characteristics of the healthy—though this is likely to become a more rewarding exercise as subtler indices of health are developed.

Special vulnerability to illness results from the possession of a number of interacting characteristics—biological, genetic, environmental, psychosocial, and so on. Thus the pregnant, the very young, the migrant, the elderly and the poor are especially vulnerable; while the young adult and the affluent are generally less so. Our ability to measure some of these risks accurately is relatively recent and provides us with the means with which to apply ourselves particularly to the preventive aspect of health care. Because of the recent emphasis on primary health care this new knowledge may have come at a specially opportune time both to increase the effectiveness of primary care and to serve the Alma-Ata ideal of health for all by the year 2000.

The possession by communities, families or individuals of characteristics which confer a special risk of disease implies some sort of causal chain or sequence, and certain of these attributes can be described easily and in detail—malnutrition, infancy, old age and pregnancy, for example. The associated risks, which can be converted into "scores" for managerial purposes, are in fact a kind of shorthand expression of the probable future need for care. Thus a pregnant woman with high blood pressure may be at a very high risk of a complicated labour, and the measured risk to her and her child is an expression of her need for help—that is, for preventive and curative care now. Making some estimate of the risk that, for example, the child will suffer perinatal death (a first step in the risk approach), however accurately this is done, is therefore only a signal or indicator of the extent of the woman's need. The so-called "risk strategy", which starts with these signals—these estimates of the mother's need for help—uses them as guides to action, to resource reallocation, to better coverage and referral and to family and clinical care. This is the simple and classic use of the risk approach utilizing data derived mainly from the study of individuals.

But there are also collective, community risks—for example, from the presence of malaria or schistosomiasis in a region, from air pollution or a poor water supply, and from poverty or poor health care services. The degree of risk in these cases is also an expression of need, of which the measurement is an essential component in the formation of policies—for example, in the determination of priorities and in the allocation of scarce resources. These are some of the new uses of the risk approach.

The hypothesis on which the risk approach rests, therefore, is that the more accurate these measures of risk are the more clearly will the need for help be understood, and the better (or more effective) will be the response. The risk approach applied to the individual is by no means a new concept, but its use as a policy and managerial tool is, and this tool has become sharper with the improvement of methods of measuring risk and with the increasing wealth of information available.

The ethical imperative of the equitable provision of care requires that special attention should be paid by the community and its services[1] to inequalities in health, to specially vulnerable groups and, within these groups, to those at higher risk. Such attention should also help in the more efficient use of scarce resources for care and cure as well as prevention. It will also discriminate positively in the sense of providing more care for those in need and, where possible, *in proportion to that need*. This, too, is a new aspect of the risk approach. The purpose of this book is to elaborate these hypotheses and the notion of positive discrimination in the attack on inequalities in health, and to suggest a strategy which might be tested by health systems research or by personal experience. Such a strategy depends on the measurement of risk and the ability to predict.

1.2 Preventive Medicine Becomes More Numerate

The study of a small number of representative cohorts of births,[2] and of occupational and other groups over long periods has made possible the more accurate linking of the characteristics of these groups to a variety of health outcomes, thus allowing early and more or less accurate predictions to be made.

These characteristics, measured directly or by proxy, are referred to as risk factors and the strength of the association with the outcome is

---

[1] As will be shown below, this includes the idea of self and family attention.
[2] See, for example, the report on the 1958 British Perinatal Mortality Survey (*1*).

known as the relative risk (see section 3.3.2). Estimation of the chances of an adverse outcome when one or more risk factors are present, measurement of their interaction as predictors, and calculations of what might happen to the health of the population if the risk factors were removed make possible a number of applications in preventive medicine. These risks, predictions and possible effects are therefore the tools of the risk approach.[1] They must be examined in each case to determine which are of the most value, and it remains to be seen which is worth using and which is too cumbersome or as yet too inaccurate or expensive of resources for general use. The new uses of data must, of course, be the subject of careful scrutiny; this is the research which *must* precede the "prescriptive" or general application of the risk approach.

Behind this need for support from data before a widespread use is contemplated lies a more general philosophy. It is that *any* increase in our knowledge of the frequency and severity of unmet health care needs in the community can only lead to a greater concern for the more rational and effective use of health care resources; such an improvement in knowledge is likely to alert families and services to what will have to be done. Even in the extreme example of terminal illness, increased concern and knowledge will probably lead to more effective care. What is not known without careful research is how much more efficient and effective such a process is than health care without the use of the risk data.[2]

The principles of the risk approach are generally applicable, but special attention is at present being directed to the problems of the most vulnerable of population groups—namely, mothers and children. Training programmes in the appropriate health systems research methods are under way. In the meantime there is a need for a more realistic approach to priority health problems, particularly in the poorer areas of the world—one that will have as its objective the direction of existing and potential resources to those in greatest need and the increase of the effectiveness of primary health care. In the development of these local plans the risk concept may be of value; its general purpose may be stated as follows:

By quantifying the risks to the health of a population and their associated risk factors it focuses attention on the need for prevention.

This information can then be used in a variety of contexts—in the home, in the community, in the clinic and hospital, and in local training programmes and policy development.

In order to gather and to use this information it will be necessary to:

---

[1] These "tools" are new only in the sense that they comprise new data; some of their uses have been known for many years. They are described in detail in section 2.3, p. 15 et seq.
[2] Even the most simple and apparently straightforward of preventive measures may involve hazards. Great care must be taken to ensure that no damage follows an apparent improvement (see section 3.5).

(1) measure the risk of maternal and child health problems occurring in the community and provide some kind of mechanism for surveillance of both population and services which will show how well the problems are being prevented and whether the interventions are beneficial or otherwise;

(2) make predictions regarding the level of care required by individuals or communities at different levels of risk;

(3) provide anticipatory care and allocate resources to individuals and groups at different levels of risk, in proportion to that risk;

(4) increase popular knowledge of risk and risk factors so that the risk approach may be more generally used, especially in the home and the community; and

(5) present the risk data in such a way as to facilitate their use in the planning and evaluation of health care, including intersectoral contributions.

In later chapters an attempt is made to illustrate with specific and simple examples some of the ways in which risk information might be used to strengthen primary health care.

1.3 The Risk Approach and the Contribution of Health Services

Much effort by governments and international nongovernmental agencies has gone into the improvement of health services in both developed and developing countries. Despite considerable progress, there remain many areas of the world where access to such services is limited to less than a quarter of the population. These massive gaps in care and associated inequalities in health—often much greater within countries than between them—have helped to overemphasize the contribution which health services can make to health. Often this is at the expense of giving due recognition to other important determinants of health and illness, which are outside the formal health care system. In the past, it was reasonable for many policy-makers as well as most health professionals to believe that the provision of *medical* care, especially up-to-date hospital care, would ensure the good health of the populations served. Challenged by Illich (2), McKeown (3), and others, this oversimplified assumption has lost credence, and there is now a real danger that opinion will swing in the opposite direction—almost to a rejection of the value of formal health care as a major factor in community health.

Three facts have emerged from the controversy and from the conciliatory studies of Martini et al. (4), among other writers. Each is relevant to the application of the risk approach to health care. First, and not surprisingly, health care of any kind—but particularly care at the primary level—seems to contribute to health roughly in proportion to the local unmet health needs. This means that in the face of great need even a small improvement in the provision of health care to a neighbourhood (such as that which might be expected from the application of the risk approach) is likely to result in a disproportionate improvement in health. If the neighbourhood already enjoys a reasonable level of health the contribution will be proportionately less. Secondly, the effect of health care services on health will, of course, depend to a great extent on the local problems and the indices used to measure them. Some indices—perinatal mortality, for example—are more sensitive than others to the impact of health care. Finally, it seems likely that in some cultures the more subjective the description of health—that is, the more it reflects local feelings rather than merely pathological findings—the more it will be influenced by health care services, especially if they are accepted and correspond to the beliefs and values of the population. As will be seen below, formal health care innovations based on the use of risk are designed to be used where the need is great, with indices which respond to formal and informal health care and which pay much attention to local values and priorities. So while it is not expected that the risk approach will at once produce a healthy population, there seems sufficient justification for using it, especially where the need for care is great.

Other contributions to the health of populations derive, of course, from genetic, environmental, socioeconomic and educational factors, as well as from social and family support systems. Measures of risk, by linking these factors to outcomes—however crudely—may direct attention to the need for changes in resource allocation, social services or lifestyle for both community and individual. This could be done by allotting a measure of the "blame" (or a proportion of the total risk) to risk factors such as poor social support, illiteracy, poverty, and malnutrition—that is, to "causes" outside the formal health care system (5). While there are problems of method in this kind of analysis which need to be dealt with,[1] the approach may gain in importance as the potential of intersectoral contributions to the health of communities becomes increasingly recognized.

1.4 Predicting Health

Improvements in our ability to predict illness and death have raised once more the problem of the prediction—using the risk factor model—of health. Classic definitions do not help us, for, at the present time and from a statistical point of view, health is clearly the absence of definable disease and a low risk of future disease. However, there are on the research horizon a number of measures of wellbeing and "quality of life"

---

[1] The attributable risk has great potential (see Foreword) and may be of increasing value in policy formulation (see section 3.3.3).

(6), and their associations are being studied. With their development, the possibility is emerging of an analogue of the risk approach to disease—a series of interacting factors which together can be used to predict something more than low risk: the chance of achieving positive wellbeing and a high quality of life. That these concepts should be incorporated into the risk approach to primary health care is essential, and more research is needed.

2. Promoting the health of mothers and children

2.1 The Risk Approach Applied to Maternal and Child Health

Of all population groups, mothers and children are the most susceptible to good or harmful influences that will permanently affect their health. Moreover, the harm can be inflicted or the "good" promoted in a very short time. The effects are long-term and "intergenerational," and there is also an influence on adult health. This extreme sensitivity of the young family—i.e., the mother and father and their young children—to all kinds of health intervention has long been recognized. What has not been so widely appreciated, however, are the special implications for the young family of the new emphasis on primary health care (7). This part of the population is so susceptible, as far as its state of health is concerned, that it is more likely than any other group to be affected by variations in the quality of the care which it uses most—that is, primary care.

Of all the components of primary health care[1] those which have the greatest impact are, of course, the ones which include promotion and prevention. For this reason any new approaches in these directions will show their greatest "yield" in the improved health of the young family; it will not only be the main recipient but the chief beneficiary as well.

Community awareness of the special vulnerability of the young family has led to the popular recognition of risk factors. For example, late or early reproductive age, poverty, maternal malnutrition, poor birth spacing, history of intercurrent illness, high parity and a host of other indicators of risk are, in many cultures, well recognized as the hazards of pregnancy. Some of the causal pathways are understood and have led to local uses of the risk idea.

There would seem to be no reason why this popular recognition should not be extended to risk factors beyond pregnancy. If this were so, the whole of maternal and child health could benefit from the economy of such an approach to promotion and prevention—particularly the use

---

[1] The eight components of primary health care are described in the report of the Alma-Ata conference (8).

of risk factors which can predict interruptions to normal growth and development.

The challenge presented by more accurate knowledge thus consists in how best to use this "epidemiology of risk", how to exploit more of the known causal pathways, and how to improve—even slightly—the effectiveness of prevention (and, of course, promotion) in the domain of maternal and child health care and family planning.[1] Essentially this is a problem of how to enhance and improve the coverage, acceptability, efficiency and the effectiveness of primary health care.

2.2 Health Problems and the Concepts of Risk and Chance

2.2.1 Risk

Risk implies that the probability of adverse consequences is increased by the presence of one or more characteristics or factors. Risk is thus a measure of statistical chance, the probability of a future occurrence—usually undesired (see, for example, reference 9). When the probability of the occurrence of a disease, illness, accident or death can be reduced or nullified if anticipatory action is taken, then this action uses the risk approach at an individual level.

The notion of risk is widely understood, particularly when applied to games, though in the context of personal or family health it may be alarming (10). Knowledge of the likelihood of a future event may be rendered less frightening if the chances of avoiding that event are understood. Risk of disease is also less likely to provoke anxiety if the notion is used to indicate the skills that are needed to prevent the disease and to promote health.

2.2.2 Luck and chance

If the risk of, say, perinatal death among the entire population between the gestational age of 28 weeks and the end of the first week of life were on average 100 per 1000, a detailed study of the distribution of such risk would reveal that it was anything but equal for all that population. Some would have a very high risk of death (the method of predicting which individuals constitute this group and what action should be taken are the subject of this book), while others would have a very low risk. None would have no risk, while many would have a moderate risk. Fig. 1[2] shows this distribution with a hypothetical curve illustrating how different risks are to be found in a population of

---

[1] The planning of families, though usually thought of in terms of birth-spacing and number of children, has much wider connotations, including that of the planning of the whole of family life.

[2] A set of colour slides, suitable for teaching purposes, based on the figures and tables in this book may be purchased from Distribution and Sales, World Health Organization, 1211 Geneva 27, Switzerland.

Fig. 1. A distribution of risk

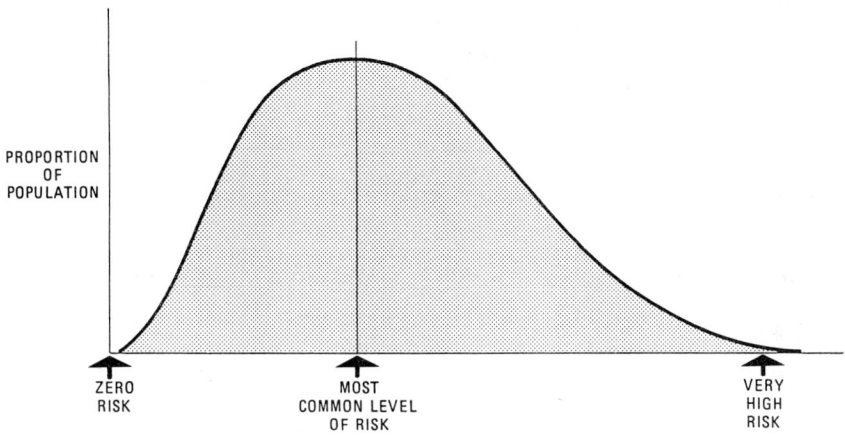

Notes: Different communities will have different distributions of risk.

No one has zero risk.

mothers. Even among those mothers with a very high risk of their children dying there will be many whose offspring will survive, and, likewise, among those children most likely to survive there will be a few deaths. A scrutiny of the records after the event often points to causes which suggest that the risks were wrongly estimated but, even after that scrutiny, there will be unforeseen survivors among those at very high risk and unforeseen deaths among those with the lowest risk. The risk approach involves the assumption that as knowledge increases so these unforeseen events will become fewer and fewer. But in the meantime it is important to recognize that not all events can be "explained" and chance still plays a part.[1] While we can estimate roughly how many will die in a given population in a given period, we cannot predict with accuracy which individuals will die.

2.2.3 Risk factors

A risk factor has been defined as any ascertainable characteristic or circumstance of a person or group of persons that is known to be associated with an abnormal risk of developing or being especially adversely affected by a morbid process.[2] Our own definition is that a risk factor is one link in a chain of associations leading to an illness—or an indicator of a link.

---

[1] Technically, not all the variance can be explained and some of what is left is a chance variation. This notion is discussed by A. J. Ayer (*11*) and by Doll & Peto (*12*).

[2] WHO Regional Office for Europe. *Symposium on the identification of high risk persons and population groups, Windsor, 1972*, Copenhagen, 1973 (unpublished document EURO 4911).

Risk factors can therefore be causes or signals but the important thing about them is that they are observable or identifiable *prior* to the event they predict. Risk factors may characterize the individual, the family, the group, the community, or the environment. Several studies have shown that first pregnancy, high parity, pregnancy at early or late reproductive age, close spacing of births, previous child loss, and malnutrition are universal risk factors which increase the chance of a poor outcome of pregnancy. Combinations of these and other risk factors in the same individual further raise the chance of a poor outcome. Moreover, the interaction of biological risk factors with others derived from the social and environmental setting will have an increased effect. For example, multiparity in mothers living in poverty is associated with a higher risk of a perinatal death than multiparity on its own.[1]

Risk factors are therefore characteristics which have a significant association with a defined outcome. It is important to specify the outcome for which each risk factor or combination of factors is sought. For example, the term "infant death" is not detailed enough, because the characteristics of mothers whose infants have an increased chance of dying from hypoxia during delivery, for instance, may be quite different from those of mothers whose infants die from gastroenteritis.

Risk factors may be specific to a particular outcome, such as a previous induced abortion leading to cervical incompetence. More frequently, however, one risk factor increases the chances of a number of outcomes or end-points perhaps to quite a different extent. An example is grand multiparity, with its increased risk of several complications of pregnancy and delivery, such as transverse lie, antepartum haemorrhage, and premature and precipitate birth (see Fig. 2A).

It has been emphasized that risk factors are characteristics of individuals or their environment that have a statistical association with the defined outcome. Except for rare, dominant, inherited disease, the statistical association between risk factor and outcome is far from absolute. For example, smoking during pregnancy carries a risk of increasing perinatal mortality from 20 to 30 per 1000, according to one study (*13*). However, over 90% of pregnant smokers have healthy surviving babies, albeit of lower-than-average birth weight.

The significance of the risk factor to preventive medicine depends not only on the extent of the association with the outcome, but also on the frequency of the risk factor in the community. If a certain risk factor were to carry a high probability of, say, fetal death, this would be of considerable importance to the mother concerned. However, if this risk factor were uncommon in the community, the impact on the *total* fetal mortality experienced by that community would be small (see section

---

[1] The selection of a combination of risk factors with optimum predictability and the avoidance of "overlapping" factors involve complex arithmetic. The method is described in a workbook, which is available, on request, from the Division of Family Health, World Health Organization, Geneva, Switzerland. (See also section 2.2.5.)

Fig. 2A. **The relationship between risk factors and outcomes: three risk factors and one outcome**

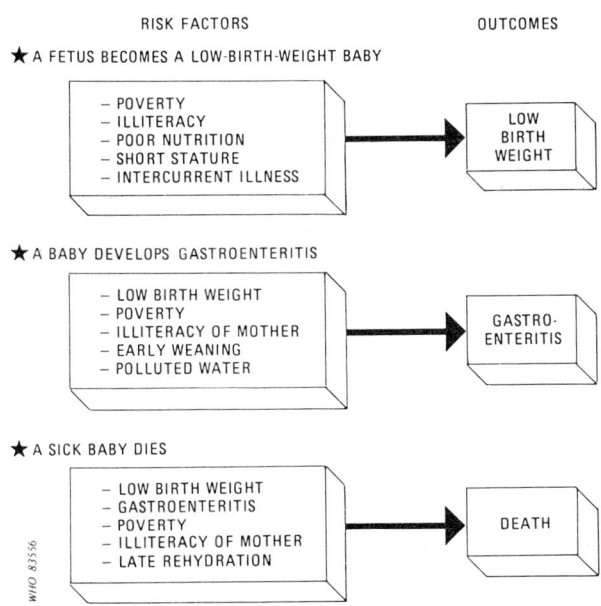

3.3.3) and this fact would have to be considered when control policies were framed.

2.2.4 Risk factors and causes

In almost all societies links are popularly recognized between the outcome of pregnancy and preceding events. These are often held to be causal though they may depend only on temporal associations, which are notoriously misleading. It must be remembered that events which precede other events do not necessarily cause them. Only in some communities is this principle accepted, and rarely in those where childbirth is surrounded by folklore and deeply entrenched beliefs in magic.

The notion of "cause" is complex (*14*), and not all significant associations between the characteristics of the vulnerable and the unwanted outcome are part of a chain of causality. Some of the most useful are statistical only. Associations are usually described as "causal" if they can be seen to be directly related to pathological processes, even if the pathways are not fully understood. Examples include maternal malnutrition and low birth weight, placenta praevia and fetal death from anoxia, or first-trimester rubella and congenital malformations.

The criteria which strongly suggest a "causal" association between risk factor and outcome are the *strength*, or "power", of the factor concerned in the statistical sense (see Chapter 3); whether there is a "*dose-response relationship*"—that is, whether, as the characteristic increases or decreases, the outcome becomes more or less frequent; its *specificity*, or the uniqueness of the relationship;[1] its *time relationship*; its *consistency*, or the repeatability of the observations; and, finally, its *biological plausibility* (though here we must be careful not to reject some of the traditional wisdom embodied in folklore).

Recognition of risk factors which are part of the causal chain of events leading to illness or death (the unwanted outcome) is the more challenging, since intervention will often lower the risk (see section 5.3.4). In instances where risk factors are still strictly part of the causal chain of events, such as high maternal age or previous fetal or child loss, but where intervention to alter the pathology is either impossible or not understood, a different response is called for—one that is *compensatory*. This would entail the alerting of services and ensuring that their state of preparedness is in proportion to the risk involved.

Finally, there are risk factors, sometimes with impressive predictive power, such as poverty or crowding or membership of a particular ethnic group, where associations only reflect the causal pathways. Others are even more distant from pathology but may still be useful indicators. Thus if a family lacks a means of transport, such as a bicycle, or its housing is of poor quality (readily ascertainable risk factors), this is indicative of a group of interacting forces (the most important of which is probably poverty) that expose an expectant mother in that family to a high risk, the degree of which can be estimated.

The attribution of "cause" to a risk factor will therefore only be of importance in helping to define what action to take. The statistically determined degree of risk associated with a risk factor may, however, be equally useful as a predictor of outcome whether this arises from pathology or some apparently unconnected indicator of risk such as the examples cited above.

Risk factors are therefore ascertainable indicators of what is going on inside a complex interacting biological and social system and the definition as well as the understanding of "causes" within this system is necessarily limited.[2] The precise "causes" of poor pregnancy outcome among those with previous fetal or child loss, therefore, are not always clear, though the risk is. Not all the factors which predispose a toddler to an excessive number of accidents if the mother works outside the home are understood, though in some cultures outside work is a significant risk factor. Another common example is the association between poverty and infant gastroenteritis, where the complex of poverty

---

[1] This is not a good criterion since so many characteristics, such as age or smoking, are not specific yet they are related causally to many unwanted outcomes.

[2] It is unusual to calculate attributable risk without direct evidence of cause. Many of the uses of risk data in sociopolitical policy formulation depend on such evidence. Thus if people with telephones have (on average) better health than those without, a more equitable distribution of telephones will not promote health—but a more equitable distribution of wealth might do so.

may include contributions to risk from large families, crowding, early weaning and poor nutrition, with infection of the infant and neglect of early diarrhoea for a variety of reasons—economic, social and cultural. Even without elucidating the pathways of causation, it is clear that family poverty is a risk factor for gastroenteritis in the infant; it is probably an even more important risk factor for death from gastroenteritis (see Fig. 2B).

The chain of events which takes an infant from health to death from gastroenteritis appears to be a linear progression from poverty through ignorance and illiteracy, low birth weight, early weaning, infection, rehydration administered too late or not at all, to marasmus and death. This notion of a chain or sequence, though it highlights risk factors and prompts intervention at each stage, obscures the fact that what is happening is part of a much more complex system of interactions. Not only are there many other contributions (some additive and some synergistic) but many of the risk factors can also be regarded as outcomes and the risks of the next step change as the sequence advances.

Medical care in the past has concentrated on associations where the pathological processes could be interrupted. This preoccupation has led to neglect of the more tenuous links in the causal chain, which, like

Fig. 2B. The relationship between risk factors and outcomes: an outcome can also be a risk factor

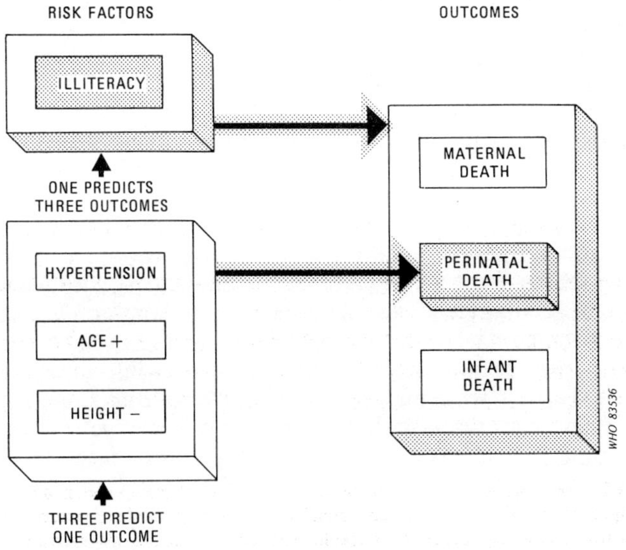

Notes: This is only a selection of possible risk factors.

Combinations of risk factors have complex relationships (see section 2.2.5).

poverty, are difficult "nonmedical" challenges. One feature of the use of the risk approach is that it prompts attention to all "causes" regardless of their medical, intersectoral, emotional, political, economic or even occult origins. The notion of risk thus forces attention to factors that are remote links in the orthodox chain of causality—beyond poverty to the causes of poverty, beyond undernutrition to the economics of food distribution, beyond low birth weight to community attitudes to women. The risk approach cannot, of course, unravel all these associations but may go some way to defining their relative importance.

2.2.5 Combinations of risk factors

The association between the risk factor, indicator or signal of a future event and the outcome itself is most easily studied where only one risk factor predicts one outcome—for example, the possession of a motorized bicycle by an adolescent boy and the risk of accident, a history of hypertensive disease in pregnancy and perinatal or maternal death, or maternal malnutrition and low birth weight. However, the combination of two or more risk factors—for example, hypertensive disease plus poor prenatal care—usually makes perinatal death more likely. The converse is also true—a single powerful risk factor may be used to predict a number of unwanted outcomes (see Fig. 2A). The selection of combinations of risk factors with maximum predictive power is important but complicated; it is partly a statistical and partly an operational problem (see section 3.4.1).

2.2.6 Communities at risk

High-risk communities have received less attention than high-risk individuals, but there is historical evidence of a concern for community groups. One such example is the observation that residents of certain areas were more exposed to "fevers" at certain seasons, which dates back to Hippocrates. Another is Ramazzini's documenting the increased risk of disease in defined occupational groups at the end of the 17th century; yet another is William Farr's demonstration, nearly 140 years ago, of increased mortality among residents of large English cities, the rate being at its highest in certain boroughs of London. Today, migrants living in the shanty towns of many cities are at a greater risk of tuberculosis and sexually transmitted diseases, while every country has its depressed areas with higher infant mortality and morbidity. A high prevalence of the same risk factors, such as type of employment, socioeconomic class or characteristics of residence, can thus be associated with the added risk of death or disease for groups of individuals, regardless of their individual susceptibilities.

The possibility of identifying those at risk by group characteristics and of calculating their risks, without the need to contact individuals, may be used in planning interventions; the method is referred to in Chapter 5.

2.3 The Potential of the Risk Approach

The risk approach involves, first, decisions as to priority "targets", or unwanted outcomes, measurement of associations between risk factors and outcomes, and then intervention planned in such a way that it makes best use of the measurements in the context of local cultures and formal and informal health care. Next comes the evaluation of these innovations and their modification before wider application. This can be part of a routine service, or a research programme,[1] or both. The difference is not in the approach, for both types are asking questions and seeking answers, but in the rigour of the evaluation and in design.

Whether they take the form of a service or of a research programme, applications of the risk approach will lean on a number of crucial measurements which can be referred to as "the tools of the risk approach". The patterns they make constitute the epidemiology of risk in the region concerned. The structure of health care systems (and indeed the structure of local and national government) will determine which part can benefit from their use. A clear distinction must be observed between the derivation of risk measures, which is often complex, and their use, which should be simple, particularly at the level of the care of the individual.

Perhaps the most important tool of the risk approach is an attitude of mind which sees estimates of risk as estimates of the urgency of need for promotive, preventive and early curative care and the prevalence of

Table 1. Perinatal death rates in four high-risk groups: all births, Cuba, 1973

Risk factors	% of all births	Perinatal mortality per 1000 births				
		Late fetal	Congenital anomaly	Immaturity	Obstetric causes	All causes
Mother parity 4+	18.1	26.8	1.9	1.2	5.5	40.4
Mother's age under 18 years	9.1	11.4	1.6	2.5	4.2	30.7
Mother single	35.8	16.3	..	..	..	32.8
Non-hospital delivery	3.5	22.4	..	..	..	40.9
All mothers	100.0	12.8	1.4	1.6	4.0	26.9

Source: World Health Organization. *Social and biological effects on perinatal mortality*, Budapest, Statistical Publishing House, 1978.

Notes: .. = not available.
"Late fetal" deaths includes some deaths from the other, more specific, causes.

---

[1] The workbook that forms the basis of WHO-supported training workshops (see footnote[1], page 10) is concerned with the different study designs which can be used in innovation and evaluation.

Table 2. Some uses for risk information: perinatal death rates in four high-risk groups, all births, Cuba, 1973

Prevalence of risk factors: use in social policy, community and intersectoral action

Relative risk: use for scoring, referral, community and family education, individual priority setting, resource allocation, etc.

Attributable risk for priority setting and policy development

Absolute risk associated with each risk factor: use in evaluation, community and family education and in alerting the health care system

Risk for the whole population: use in priority setting, planning services, etc. Shows the size of the problem

Incidence data can be used in task analyses, priorities for training and in clinical strategies

The risk factors themselves are guides to preventive medicine

Risk factors	% of all births	Perinatal mortality per 1000 births					Relative risk	Attributable risk (%)
		Late fetal	Congenital anomaly	Immaturity	Obstetric causes	All causes		
Mother parity 4+	18.1	26.8	1.9	1.2	5.5	40.4	1.69	11
Mother's age under 18 years	9.1	11.4	1.6	2.5	4.2	30.7	1.16	2
Mother single	35.8	16.3	...	...	...	32.8	1.39	12
Non-hospital delivery	3.5	22.4	...	...	...	40.9	1.54	1
All mothers	100.0	12.8	1.4	1.6	4.0	26.9	1.00	—

Note: ... = not available.

WHO 83601

risk in the population as a challenge to make optimum use of appropriate skills and technologies.

There are many ways in which societies promote the health of their mothers and children, and this book considers how the addition of risk data (the tools of the risk approach) might be of assistance. However, the risk approach is no panacea: it is rather a series of suggestions for the exploitation of this information and these ideas in different parts of formal and informal health care systems. New health problems are constantly presenting themselves and each one demands new solutions. To some of these the risk approach already provides insights. New kinds of vulnerability arise—for example, that of adolescents, which stems from striking contemporary demographic trends and the breakup of the extended family, the urban drift of young migrants, the loneliness, unemployment and increasing threats from accidents, violence, smoking and drug and alcohol abuse. The associated risks and risk factors may be roughly quantified and this quantification will help to achieve an understanding of the relevant chain of events and thus perhaps aid prevention. Tables 1 and 2 illustrate (with data now some years old) how even limited information about risk might be utilized. Table 1 presents a conventional tabulation of data about perinatal mortality and Table 2 presents the same material with a few simple calculations added. (Relative and attributable risks are described in Chapter 3 and their calculation is summarized in Annex 2.) Some possible uses of these data are superimposed.

3. Outcome, risk and measurement

In this chapter are described the data which are the basis of the risk approach and how they are acquired.

3.1 The Data Base

The risk approach seeks to use information about risk to prevent a variety of adverse outcomes (that is, illness, injury and death) through the application of a strategy at many levels of care. The data about risk which are needed for these different uses are enumerated below.

3.1.1 Outcomes

The first information required will usually be a list of mortality or morbidity rates (or best estimates) pertaining to certain illnesses, reductions in which could be the locally chosen targets or priorities. Ideally the rates would be age and sex specific—that is, rates for, say, 5-year age groups, and for each sex separately—and based on whole populations or on representative samples. Depending, of course, on the intended application, additional information would be of value in determining priorities and detecting risk factors. For example, a knowledge of the size of the problem (prevalence and incidence[1]) is essential for all planning; also of relevance are some socioeconomic or occupational distributions of the data and distributions by area and, perhaps, population density. Some time trends, as well as detailed information about how these outcomes or "health needs" are at present dealt with, are essential as an indicator of their importance and of the present efficacy of control.

The risk to the whole population of these outcomes (the rates per 1000) would not only indicate the size of the problem but help in the designation of group risk (see section 2.2.6 above and sections 3.3.1 and

---

[1] The *prevalence* of an illness is the number of cases in the community at any one time. The *incidence* of an illness is the number of new cases occurring in a given period. Both measures are rates—that is, the number of cases per 1000 population.

3.3.3 below). It would also be useful as a crude criterion for later evaluation.

3.1.2 Risk factors

The desired data base would also provide the following information:

(1) *For each unwanted outcome*:

—A list of risk factors classified so that those known to have pathological connexions with the outcome appear first. Also distinguished would be the most significant combinations of risk factors and the most significant risk factor.

(2) *For each group of unwanted outcomes*:

—A list of risk factors or combinations of risk factors classified as above.

(3) *For all risk factors*:

—Their prevalence and incidence in the population and their trends in time. (These data reflect patterns of "causes" of the chosen disease or fatality, or point to what must be attacked if the unwanted outcomes are to be prevented.)

—The relative risk of unwanted outcomes associated with each risk factor or combination of risk factors (see section 3.3.2, Fig. 3 and 4 and Annex 2).

—The attributable risk associated with each risk factor or combination of risk factors (see section 3.3.3, Fig. 3 and 4 and Annex 2).

—The predictive power of each risk factor or combination of risk factors.

—The proportion of "false positives" and "false negatives" (see section 3.5) to be expected and tolerated when screening for the presence of the risk factors.

—The ease, accuracy and acceptability of screening for the presence of the various risk factors in communities and individuals.

3.2 Priorities Among Outcomes

Since the application of the risk approach involves the calculation of risk as its first step, this risk must be of a defined unwanted outcome, such as maternal or infant death, adolescent pregnancy or a motorcycle accident. While in reality many unwanted outcomes are the object of the risk approach (see Chapter 5), the necessary calculations are simpler where only one unwanted outcome is the target of the approach and of the different applications which are developed. Events that are uniformly fatal but excessively rare, although of great importance to the affected individual and the family, will inevitably carry a low priority because the detection of the risk factors involved and their modification may require so many resources. This is true even in rich societies, as, for example, in the case of amniocentesis for the detection of genetic defects. Similarly, other conditions, which, though uncommon, involve the need for continuous care—e.g., spina bifida with meningomyelocele—might have a different and somewhat higher priority, depending on social pressures and available resources. Again, the prevention of a common minor disability might be of higher priority than that of a more severe but rare disability.

It is thus essential to define those outcomes—death, disability or a decline in the quality of life—requiring intervention, to measure their frequency, and to rank them in some way, depending on their importance to the local community and the possibilities of prevention and treatment. Perception of "importance" will, naturally, vary from culture to culture.

Whether only one health problem of mothers and children or the ten most important are chosen for attack, the way of thinking about priorities is essentially the same. Five principles are usually involved:

(1) Considerable weight should be accorded to community priorities, preferences and concerns.

(2) The more common problems should have a higher priority than the more rare.

(3) The more serious problems should be given higher priority than the less serious.

(4) The more easily preventable health problems of mothers and children should have a higher priority than those that are more difficult.

(5) Health problems whose frequencies show upward trends in time should in general be given higher priority than those that are static or declining.

A number of ways of combining these criteria to give an order of preference—a priority order—are available, and one is shown in Annex 1. The morbidity or mortality (the unwanted outcome) at the top of the list thus becomes the health problem at which the risk strategy will be aimed.

3.3 The Measurement of Risk

Once the unwanted outcome has been decided on and a full description of its epidemiology and of all of the risk factors involved has been obtained, the next step is the measurement of risk. In the more sophisticated research studies, cohorts of mothers and children would be followed over long periods, all the risk factors defined, and the detailed statistical and pathological nature of the associations established. In other studies it may be sufficient to use the data from research in similar cultures and surroundings, or from cross-sectional studies. Whichever course is followed, measures of risk will have to be established. This is often a formidable task involving new recording systems, but, while it is difficult to avoid the special surveys which reveal the nature and occurrence of outcomes in particular communities, some of the associated risk factors are likely to be universal. In fact it is probable that the majority of the risk factors that have been identified to date—particularly in the field of reproductive performance—are of biological significance and thus probably of general application. For perinatal mortality and morbidity, for instance, these risk factors will include early or late reproductive age, high parity, adverse maternal habits, infections, hypertension and bleeding during pregnancy, deficient availability and type of prenatal care and obstetric intervention, and lack of facilities for resuscitation and later care of the newborn. There will also be population risk factors such as poverty, a low level of parental education and intercurrent disease.

At its least complicated the risk strategy uses three measures of risk of a future illness, accident or death. All are based on incidence rates—that is, the number of new occurrences of the unwanted outcome over a given period in a given population.

3.3.1 Risk to the whole population

First, there is the risk of the unwanted outcome occurring among the whole population, which, of course, includes those with and those without definable risk factors. This is sometimes called the absolute risk. Since it expresses the actual chances of an event—the probability of the illness, accident or death occurring during a given period—it is a most valuable indicator. Thus in Table 1 (p. 15) the risk of a perinatal death for that particular community was 26.9 for every 1000 births—that is, approximately 2.7%.

3.3.2 Relative risk

Next, there is the relative risk of the outcome occurring among those with one or more risk factors. This is one of the most useful of measures and expresses the ratio between the incidence of the illness or cause of death in the population of those with the risk factor (or factors) and the corresponding incidence in the population of those without the risk factor (or factors). It is therefore a measure of the strength of the association between risk factor and outcome. Thus a relative risk of 1.3 means a 30% excess risk among those people with that particular risk factor or factors, whereas a relative risk of 3.0 means a 200% excess risk[1] (Fig. 3). It is sometimes called the "odds ratio".

---

[1] Note also that the relative risk is not an "observed"-to-"expected" ratio since the expected would represent the whole population and not only those without the risk factor. It will also be appreciated that all these measures are subject to the rules of statistical probability and have their own confidence limits, and that spurious associations and many confounding variables exist to entrap the unwary.

Fig. 3. Relative risk

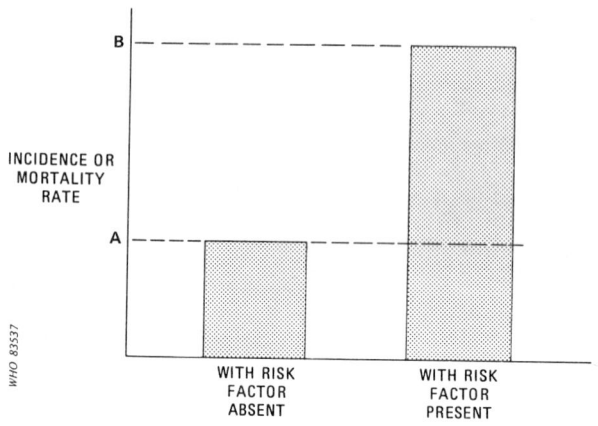

Note: The relative risk is sometimes called the "odds ratio". In the example it is $\frac{B}{A}$.

In the example of smoking during pregnancy, which was given in section 2.2.3, the occurrence of a perinatal death among the children of mothers who smoked was 30 per 1000 and among mothers who did not it was 20 per 1000. The relative risk of smoking was therefore 1.5 and the excess risk of a perinatal death among the offspring of smokers was 50%.

3.3.3 Attributable risk

While the importance of a risk factor depends to a large extent on the strength of its association with the eventual outcome, from the community's point of view it also depends on the frequency of the factor in the community. If a certain risk factor were to carry a high probability of, say, fetal death but was very rare in the community, the impact of its removal on total fetal mortality would be small. This impact on the community's experience is measured by attributable risk (15–17) (Fig. 4; see also Annex 2).

Attributable risk brings together three ideas: the frequency of the unwanted outcome when the risk factor is present, the frequency of the outcome when the risk factor is absent, and the frequency of occurrence of the risk factor in the community. It therefore indicates what might be expected to happen to the overall outcome in the community if the risk factor were removed. The importance of this concept in terms of policy-making, which will be referred to below, can hardly be exaggerated (18–20). It can be illustrated briefly by an example from the controversial field of fatal accidents to children on motorized bicycles.

Suppose that the risk factor for the fatal accidents under review was "age under 16 years" and legislation was pending which would impose

Fig. 4. Attributable risk: effect on the community of the removal of two risk factors

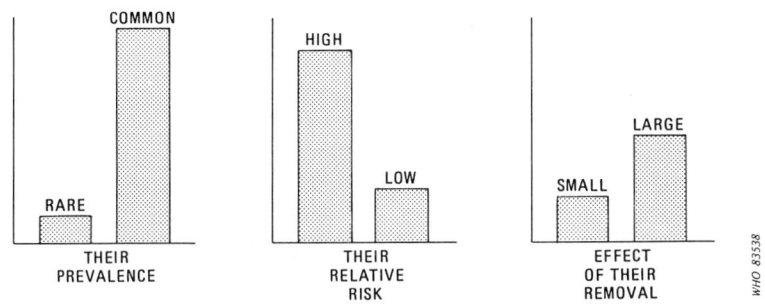

Note: Attributable risk is based on the assumption of a causal relationship between risk factor and outcome.

an age limit of 16 years, below which it would be illegal to ride a motorized bicycle. If the relative risk associated with the risk factor was 5 (or 500%)—that is, the excess risk of death associated with being under 16 years of age was 400% and the proportion of motorized cyclists below 16 years of age among all motorized cyclists was 25%— then the attributable risk, using Lilienfeld's formula (15),[1] would be 0.5, or 50%.

If the suggested change in the law were implemented (and 16 years became the minimum age for riding motorized bicycles), the most the community could expect to save (if there really were a cause-and-effect relationship and if age were independent) would be 50% of all deaths from this cause. If, in identical circumstances, the proportion of children under 16 years who had motorized bicycles among all persons with such bicycles were only 10%, the most the community could expect from the new legislation would be a drop of 28% in the mortality from motorized-bicycle accidents (see Annex 2). Unfortunately, the application of the attributable risk is rarely as clear as in this example; attribution is almost always approximate.

3.4 Identifying the Risk Factors and the Populations and Individuals at Risk

While it is logical and just to direct limited resources to those who need them, in proportion to that need, it is not easy to identify those communities and individuals who are at different levels of risk and the specific risk factors involved. The questions of how, when and where to

---

[1] The attributable risk or "etiological fraction" can be calculated by subtracting the true incidence rates when the risk factor is absent from those when it is present—if such data are available. More complicated formulae are needed to calculate attributable risk when the only data available come from study populations among whom the prevalence of the risk factors is not the same as that among the population at large. (See Annex 2.)

intervene so that risk factors can be identified, as well as who will undertake the intervention, cannot be answered dogmatically. Decisions will be influenced by the importance of local health priorities, the chains of causation relating risk factors to outcomes, the feasibility and acceptability of intervention, local and national policies, the resources available, etc. Also important in these decisions are the uses to which the risk information is to be put, and not all the tools of the risk approach will be needed for each application (21). For example, to improve referral (see section 5.3.3) risk factors for each individual must be identified and some kind of scoring system instituted. For intersectoral policy development (see section 5.3.7) the risk data that will be of use will pertain to attributable risks based on whole communities, regions or defined populations. Or again, for task analysis and the training of health care personnel, the need will be for information about the incidence and prevalence of risk factors.

It takes more effort to identify risk factors among individuals than among groups, since the former procedure requires contact with each mother and child. Screening[1] will therefore probably commence with the ascertainment of the risk factors in the population at large. If resources are limited and strategies confined to governmental and intersectoral action, the process may end there. However, some kind of screening or surveillance of the populations whose health problems are to be the target of the risk strategy is central to the whole approach. While many risk factors can be deduced from previous work in similar cultures, the relative risks derived cannot, and these must be established through local surveys—preferably (but not necessarily) longitudinal in design. The establishment of the relative risks for communities and populations depends on the availability of some kind of formal information or vital registration service. Sometimes indirect information is of great value, and some of the groups at risk of, for instance, high perinatal mortality are characterized by poor housing, overcrowding, and residence in certain neighbourhoods. Especially in urban and periurban situations, information on risk factors such as crowding, substandard housing, poor quality water supply, and deficient environmental hygiene, for instance, may be available for geographical areas and this can be used as a means of identifying populations. The following examples are cited:

(1) In one city, families that had had infants who had died of gastroenteritis were found to differ from other families by neighbourhood of residence, parental education and occupation. They did not differ from other families in their use of prenatal care or in place of delivery and type of birth attendant. A comparison of housing showed poor water and toilet facilities to be distinguishing factors associated

---

[1] Screening is a systematic review, usually of individuals, and is often a prelude to secondary—i.e., presymptomatic—prevention. Screening for the presence of risk factors is a simpler process though likely to be somewhat less accurate, for it is often prepathological as well as presymptomatic.

with high relative and attributable risk. In this example, the conclusions were that improvements in hygiene and the social environment would have a greater impact on the outcome (death from infantile gastroenteritis) than the provision of additional health care facilities.

(2) In another urban situation, there was an inverse correlation between the municipal tax level, which indicated the socioeconomic level of the neighbourhood, and the number of infants hospitalized with gastroenteritis. In this case the population subject to low municipal tax had the highest relative risk, and the tax level ("low") could be used as a risk factor for infantile disease.

Other studies have demonstrated increased risks for a number of adverse outcomes in communities of slum dwellers, migrant workers, and in inhabitants of certain areas, to name but a few of the many risk factors analysed.

3.4.1 Selection of risk factors

In order to determine which risk factors, among the many predicting the unwanted outcome, are to be used in the application of the strategy much will depend on the considerations dealt with below.

3.4.1.1 Optimum grouping

It is rare for one risk factor to be so powerful that it stands alone as a good predictor of outcome, though, when it does, its use is greatly simplified. The problem of the optimum grouping of risk factors can be solved mathematically by using various standardization techniques (*22*) (some authors simply multiply the relative risks). In the context of this book optimum combinations of risk factors will be treated as if they were one risk factor. It must be noted, however, that in choosing the combination of risk factors, operational as well as mathematical considerations are important. Unless there is a very considerable overlap between risk factors (for example, unfavourable maternal age and high parity as risk factors for perinatal death) several risk factors will give a better prediction of outcome than a single one. However, ease of identification and acceptability may be of overriding importance. Synergism (or a multiplicative relationship) between risk factors may considerably enhance their value (yield, relative risk and predictive power).

3.4.1.2 Usefulness in terms of the proposed intervention

Not only will risk factors vary in their value according to the use to which they will be put, but some uses, such as the design of health worker training programmes, will require the identification of particular kinds of risk factors for teaching purposes—for example, clinical risk factors, such as anaemia or hypertension, which it will be important to diagnose and correct. Where the risk approach is to contribute to policy formation, social, economic, and demographic risk factors would be more important, and from these the relative and attributable risks mentioned above could be calculated. Where health education is the objective, modifiable as well as easily recognizable risk factors which are familiar to the population will be more useful. Examples would derive from age, parity and previous obstetric history.

3.4.1.3 Cause and effect

For a variety of reasons (for example, the ease with which the chain of pathological events can be interrupted), the most appropriate risk factors for use with individuals will usually be those which stand in closest causal association with the unwanted outcome. These will have the highest predictive power, and a high relative risk. They will also satisfy the numerous and demanding statistical criteria involved in their definition. (The literature on this subject is extensive; see, in particular, references *15* and *18.*) For use in policy-making, community risk factors, such as poor water supply or malnutrition, are more appropriate.

3.4.1.4 Ease of modification

Risk factors, particularly those of a pathophysiological nature, such as blood pressure, that are amenable to some effective interventions are useful in the care of the individual. Immutable factors such as age and height act more as signals which, by alerting health professionals and other personnel, are of value in promoting all kinds of compensatory care, sociopolitical action such as the education of women, and health education in general.

3.4.1.5 Ease and accuracy of identification

However appropriate and discriminative it is, a risk factor must be reasonably easy to detect. For example, rhesus incompatibility, though fulfilling the first two criteria, is difficult to detect in rural communities. (The rapid development of biochemical and haematological aids which are easy to use may, however, soon make possible more complex risk assessment.) Ease of identification of risk factors is affected by the following considerations:

—the technology involved in detection and measurement: it should be simple to use, accurate and appropriate to the setting;

—the acceptability of the process of detection both to those carrying out the screening and those subjected to it: the procedure should be verbal only, or, if it involves physical examination, this should be minimal;

—the results of tests and questions: these should be easy to record and interpret;

—the repeatability and accuracy of the test for the risk factor: these should be of a high standard—that is, the inter- and intraobserver error should be small; and

—the ease with which local people can be trained to recognize the risk factor.

Thus if the risk factor under review were "a poor past obstetric history", it would be necessary, first, to describe in detail what was meant by "poor" and the extent of the inadequacy. Next, it should be asked how easily were the facts "poor" or "not poor" elicited, how acceptable was the questioning, and how often was there concordance with other observers (to detect interobserver variation). Also, one would need to know how often there was agreement with previously recorded answers by the same person (intraobserver variation). Finally, the person being interviewed might be inconsistent, and the extent and implications of such variations in recording would have to be explored and allowed for.

3.4.2 Who should do the screening?

The identification of the chosen risk factors among individual mothers and children is best attempted sequentially, the simplest steps being taken first. If the outcomes or chosen "targets" are maternal and perinatal mortality in a developing rural tropical region in which traditional birth attendants could be trained to ask about and recognize a small number of risk factors (low stature, high parity, unfavourable maternal age, poor birth spacing, history of difficult labour, etc.) the *first* screening would best be done by such workers. If resources permit, screening would be progressive in complexity and take place on three or even four subsequent occasions (Fig. 5 and 6). The latter screening

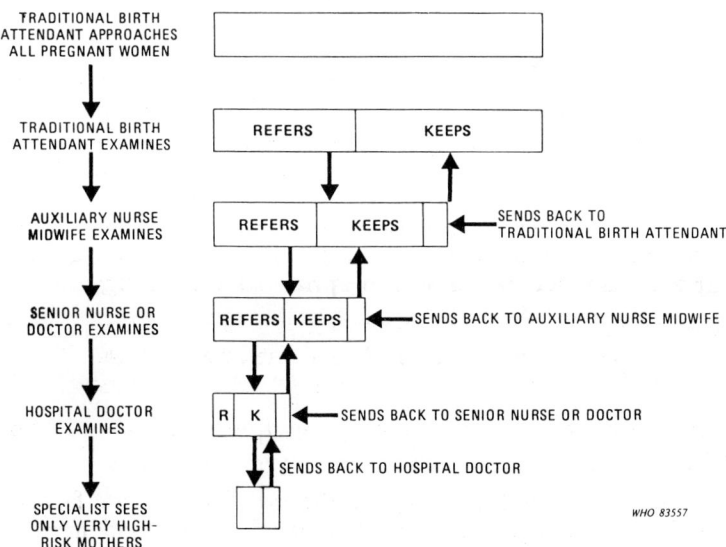

Fig. 5. The theory of screening for risk referral during pregnancy

Notes: In this example no significance is attached to population size at each step. In actuality this is dictated by a balance of resources (facilities, skills, technology, etc.) and risk.

At each step some mothers refuse further referral and some mistakes are made.

Fig. 6. Screening for risk using scores 1–5

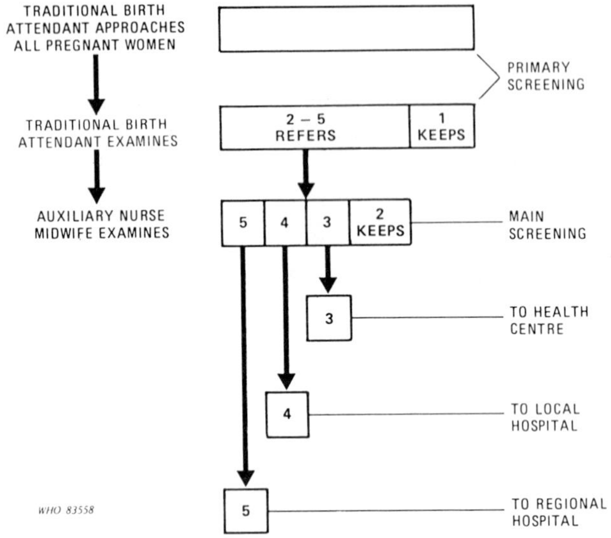

Notes: In this example no significance is attached to population size at each step. In actuality this is dictated by a balance of resources (facilities, skills, technology, etc.) and scores—reflecting risks (see section 5.3.3).

At each step some mothers refuse further referral and some mistakes are made.

would be carried out at different points along the referral chain—i.e., the sequence of persons and institutions through which an individual passes from self and family care through the formal system to the most highly organized institutions and hospitals—by increasingly skilled health personnel.

3.4.3 How should the screening be done?

The question of how to set about screening for risk at the individual level is best answered by reference to the development of simple record systems and questionnaires in association with those who will use them, and the use of appropriate technology. Local collaboration in planning the screening is necessary and two important by-products of such activity should not be overlooked. The first is that the screening of a population reverses the traditional approach to care, in which the sick seek help, coverage is probably improved (see section 5.3.2) and responsibility for initiating action lies as much with those caring as those cared for. Secondly, a large measure of community participation is called for, and if this is achieved the benefit may well spread beyond the reduction of the outcomes which are the targets of the strategy; other good and wider effects may be expected. These indirect assets, affecting local interests, attention and cooperation, are sometimes as important as the innovation itself. They are often referred to as the "Hawthorne effect".[1]

3.5 "False Positives" and "False Negatives" and Cost–Benefit Questions

When populations or, more usually, individuals are screened to find out whether they have the risk factor or factors, several kinds of difficulties of interpretation can occur. The most common and the most important are concerned with:

—whether the *presence* of the risk factor actually means that the unwanted outcome will occur, in which case the people concerned could be called "correct" or "true" positives,[2]

—whether the *absence* of the risk factor actually means that the unwanted outcome will not occur, in which case the people concerned could be called "correct" or "true" negatives.[2]

The effectiveness of the risk factor or factors at predicting the outcome will depend on the proportion of "correct" or "true" associations. An "ideal" risk factor, if present, would always be associated with the unwanted outcome and, if absent, never. However, deaths from gastroenteritis may occur among breast-fed infants (though much less commonly than among the bottle-fed), and smoking and poverty do not always predict low birth weight—and so on. So-called "false positives" and "false negatives" abound and may occur so often as to threaten clear interpretation. Table 3 illustrates two kinds of difficulties of interpretation—in this case the problem of balancing the good against the bad effects of screening for risk.

Of 225 people with the unwanted outcome in this hypothetical table the risk factor was present in 200. However, the 25 false negatives who eventually turned out to have the adverse outcome may have been neglected because of the absence of the risk factor. If the outcome had

---

[1] The term "Hawthorne effect" derives from a series of studies on scientific management in industry, which were commenced in 1924 at the Hawthorne Works of the Western Electricity Company, near Cicero, Illinois, USA, with the initial purpose of investigating the effect of illumination on productivity. Among other findings, it was discovered that the workers increased their output, not necessarily because of work changes, but because their interest was aroused by the attention that was being lavished on them. The Hawthorne effect is the expression of the concept that "novelty or interest in a new situation leads, at least initially, to positive results" (23). In the present context, this would imply that the *fact* of innovation, rather than its effects, constitutes a force for good in primary health care (see section 7.7).

[2] The proportion of all of those *with* the risk factor or factors who suffer the unwanted outcome, or, alternatively, the proportion of all of those *without* the risk factor or factors who do not suffer the unwanted outcome, represents the predictive power for that risk factor or those risk factors in the population concerned. (See Annex 2.) In Table 3 (p. 30) the predictive power of a positive test is 200/250, or 80%. The predictive power of a negative test is 725/750, or 97%.

Table 3. The balance of false positives and false negatives in the use of risk factors in preventive medicine*

Risk factor	Unwanted outcome		Totals
	Present +	Absent −	
Present +	200 true positives	50 false positives	250
Absent −	25 false negatives	725 true negatives	750
Totals	225	775	1000

* This hypothetical table is discussed further in Annex 2 and illustrated in Fig. 10 (p. 37).

been very serious (e.g., maternal mortality) this 11% would probably have been unacceptably high.[1] Of the 775 people who suffered no adverse outcome, 50 had the risk factor and their care represented some waste of resources.[2] However, this was probably quite acceptable. The real problem is: How much extra work and how many more false positives would be involved in the additional screening necessary (perhaps using other risk factors) to reduce the proportion of false negatives from 11% to acceptable levels? And what are these levels anyway? This problem and that of "trade-offs" between advantages and disadvantages is discussed in Chapter 4.

It is not easy to calculate the costs and benefits of obtaining and using the data which have been discussed. The benefits will depend on results when the information is used to improve health care, on the extent of spread of a rational approach to health care, and on the possibility of stimulating a new interest in prevention. The costs will depend largely on local factors and especially on how far they can be absorbed by the local health care system.

Difficulties are more easily described. Screening for the presence of risk factors is often inaccurate, takes time, uses many local resources (particularly human resources) and may, if done without full explanation and local participation, cause unnecessary anxiety. The risk factors that are identifiable may, for example, be complex and of low predictive

---

[1] The proportion of true positives (i.e., those with the risk factor who suffer the adverse outcome) to all those who eventually suffer the adverse outcome indicates how well the test behaved as a test of adverse outcome. This is called the sensitivity of the test. (In the example it is 200/225, or 89%.)

[2] The proportion of true negatives (i.e., those who do not suffer the adverse outcome and are without the risk factor) to all of those who eventually did not suffer the adverse outcome indicates how well the test behaved as a test of good outcome. This is called the specificity of the test. (In the example it is 725/775, or 93%.)

power, or involve too many false negatives (low sensitivity). The difficulties of collecting and analysing data in an urban slum or at village level are often underestimated. Finally, the translation of local records through coding and data analysis into usable tabulations has also presented problems.

The detection of risk factors as a prelude to prevention is probably not as costly as the biochemical testing which is its analogue in clinical care. However, since the detection procedure usually involves whole populations, it bears some similarity to presymptomatic screening for disease—though it is less haphazard—and must be treated with the same guarded and critical scrutiny before its general "prescriptive" or service use.

4. From risk measurement to intervention

4.1 Preparatory Steps

Up to this point the description of the risk approach has involved community decisions as to what are the priority problems to be tackled in promoting the health of mothers and children, in detecting risk factors and combinations of risk factors and their interrelationships, in determining their power as predictors, and in calculating the relative and attributable risks associated with them. Also known would be the incidence and perhaps prevalence of the unwanted outcomes and of the risk factors and perhaps something of their trends in time.

Before these tools of the risk approach can be used in improving the organization of health care, particularly at the individual level, three additional technical problems must be faced. A final step will be to ask whether the local health care system is able to support innovations of the kind proposed.

First—among the technical problems—an answer must be found to the question of how to convert risk data, and particularly relative risk, into simple measures which can be used at the first-contact level or at the clinic or local hospital. This is usually achieved by some form of *scoring*.

The next technical question concerns cut-off points for risk factors. This presents no problem when the risk factor is either present or absent, or where the distribution of a risk factor such as age has such sharp changes of relative risk that dichotomy or trichotomy is obvious and easy. Where, however, the distribution is continuous, the often opposing considerations of "yield" and of resources to deal with that yield impose constraints on the risk approach. (There is, for example, little advantage in a strategy which classifies 80 % of women as being at "very high risk" unless massive resources are available.)

The third technical problem is that of "trade-offs" in screening for risk. By this is meant the often painful decisions which hinge on, for example, how many false positives are to be tolerated in order to reduce the numbers of false negatives to acceptable proportions. Essentially this is the question (mentioned above) of how many and what kind of "mistakes" we can accommodate in preventive medicine and how accurate we have to be.

4.1.1 Scoring

The scoring of risk in maternal and child health, including family planning, is an attempt to provide a simple and easy-to-use index of the urgency, seriousness and complexity of the future threat to health. Scores must accurately reflect the risk to mothers and children, which in itself is a proxy for the individual's need for preventive care. Scores should group together all those at equal risk or in equal need even if the causes of that need are not the same. Thus, on a 5-point scale a "good" scoring system would select accurately, or at "5", the mothers and children whose need for preventive care (or, if an unwanted outcome was inevitable, some compensatory care) was higher than that of all the rest (see Fig. 7).

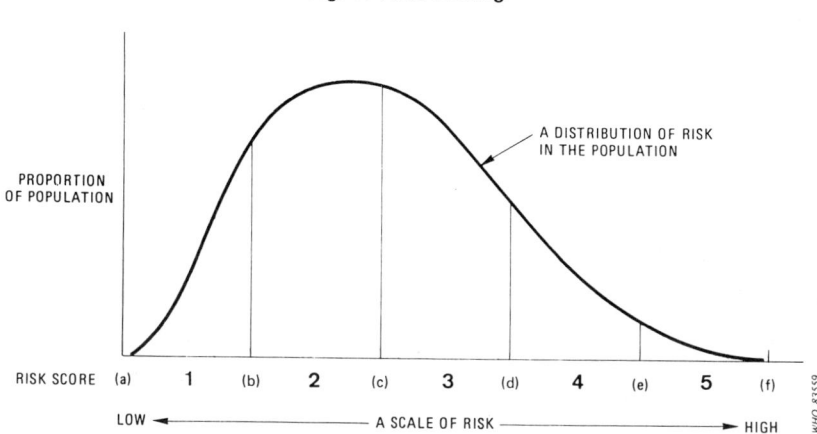

Fig. 7. Risk scoring

Note: Risks are assembled into 5 arbitrary groups in this example, so that relative risks that lie between (a) and (b) score 1, those between (b) and (c) score 2, and so on. Many other scoring arrangements are possible: all serve to link risk to skills, facilities and technology and thus facilitate preventive referral.

Risk scores are commonly used as managerial tools in maternal and child health[1] and there are four sources of such scores which should be considered. The first and most common is the *ad hoc* system, which was the earliest in use. For example, in the early work of Dugald Baird in Aberdeen, mothers were either poor (with increased risk of a bad pregnancy outcome) or not, tall (good) or short (bad), having their first child under 18 (bad) or between 18 and 26 (good), well fed or malnourished, and so on. Biochemical and blood-pressure variables were handled in much the same way and the interventions which resulted from this simple scoring were surprisingly effective, in spite of the fact

---

[1] It is worth noting that a number of senior workers with experience of scores are of the opinion that, rather than cause worry to the mother, referral to a destination compatible with a particular score is preferable to what amounts to labelling.

that only the most limited interactions between risk factors were considered. Physicians were alerted to the need for special care by the use of dichotomous risk factors. In another example the number of points or score for each risk factor is based on experience. For example, in scoring for "poor outcome" of pregnancy the PAHO/WHO system[1] allocated up to 3 points for a poor medical and/or obstetric history, up to 3 for high parity, and up to 2 for maternal age (very young or very old). Additional single points were awarded if the birth interval was short, the family income low, or the woman unmarried and of poor education. Women who obtained 6 or more points out of a total of a possible 12 were designated "high risk", while those with a score of 2 or less were termed "low risk". This and other *ad hoc* systems are of use in calling attention to women who may need special care in a given area and in guiding the decisions of primary health workers. In other areas or cultures the weight of the risk factors may be different and require the allocation of different scores.

The same *ad hoc* scoring principle has been proposed in one developing country to guide the primary health worker in referring pregnant women to the midwife. Four points are given to women under 19 or over 40, 2 to those aged 30–39, and none to those aged 20–29. Similarly, women who have had 10 or more children receive 4 points, and primiparae receive 1 point. Further points are given for short intervals between deliveries, a poor medical or obstetric history and a low educational level. If the total number of points amounts to 5 or more, the patient must be referred. In the case of 3–4 points, referral is recommended *when feasible.* This implies that the referral policy will have to be determined locally and in accordance with local resources.

The next source of information about risk and on which a risk score could be based is the absolute risk, or actual chance of illness or death where a risk factor is involved. In Table 2 (p. 16), the column headed "All causes" indicates the perinatal death rates for individuals with one of the four risk factors listed. The risk scoring of the mothers could be based on this absolute risk. For many purposes such a score would be valuable (for example, in some aspects of health education or in alerting health professionals to the actual chances of a perinatal death under each of the circumstances listed). However, the absolute risk does not immediately indicate the difference between those with and those without the risk factor, and this is done by the relative risk—the most commonly used source of risk scores. Relative risk distribution can be readily translated into simple scores, as in Fig. 7, or more complex additive or multiplicative systems can be used. Thus, in a recent study, a scoring system for women whose children were at risk of stillbirth and neonatal death resulted in the giving of 2 points for age 40 or over, 5 points for a previous stillbirth, and 1.5 points for the presence of a

---

[1] Prindle, R. A. & Gomez, C. J. *Identification of maternal risk by the PAHO/WHO system*, Washington, DC, PAHO/WHO, 1973, (unpublished document).

uterine scar from previous Caesarian sections—these figures being based on the actual relative risks without the interactions having been calculated. An even more accurate approach would be the allocation of scores based on the relative risks of combinations of risk factors, which are related as closely as possible to the defined outcome. Methods such as the analysis of variance have been used to derive such standardized scores, which are then combined, for each set of factors, to give an overall estimate of relative risk. The value of scores obtained from such analyses may not be very different from those derived more simply (for example, by adding the relative risks), although this is unlikely. There is, as yet, no good objective evidence from studies in the field of maternal and child care of a considerable increase in value due to the use of the more sophisticated measures.

The final source of risk information which might be used for scoring is the attributable risk. This invaluable guide to health policy results in a measure which is already a percentage score. That is, it indicates what percentage of the unwanted outcome being experienced by that community might be expected to disappear with the removal of the related risk factor. It would seem, therefore, that little of value is to be derived from converting attributable risks to other scores.

Most scoring systems use the relative risk; however, a WHO working group on methods of multifactor preventive trials in ischaemic heart disease[1] used an *ad hoc* scoring method for defining the top 10% of risks (the high-risk group) in the male population under study. The purpose of this scoring was, of course, quite different from any attempt to improve referral throughout a health care system. However, on analysis, the crude scores were shown to have, *for this purpose*, much the same predictive power as more sophisticated approaches. The working group nevertheless felt that more work needed to be done to develop methods of scoring. This is particularly pertinent where the actions to be taken on the basis of the scores are more complex than those in the heart disease study. There must be further experiment with different ways of providing scores and risk estimates, based on known values, for combinations of characteristics (e.g., advanced age and high parity with poor obstetric history), to test the usefulness of different ways of combining risk factors. Whatever the method chosen, the scores are only useful to the degree that they permit the accurate prediction of high-risk groups and outcomes in the future and discriminate between levels of risk.

Some workers insist that scores are of most use if they simply reflect relative risk and are not modified unless the risks which they reflect are themselves modified. Others see scores as the final tools of preventive strategies and expect them to be modified by local values and priorities, by local concepts of what is serious, and, above all, by local resources.

---

[1] WHO Regional Office for Europe. *Methodology of multifactor preventive trials in ischaemic heart disease. Report on a working group . . . , Innsbruck, 1973*, Copenhagen, 1973 (unpublished document EURO 8202 (6)).

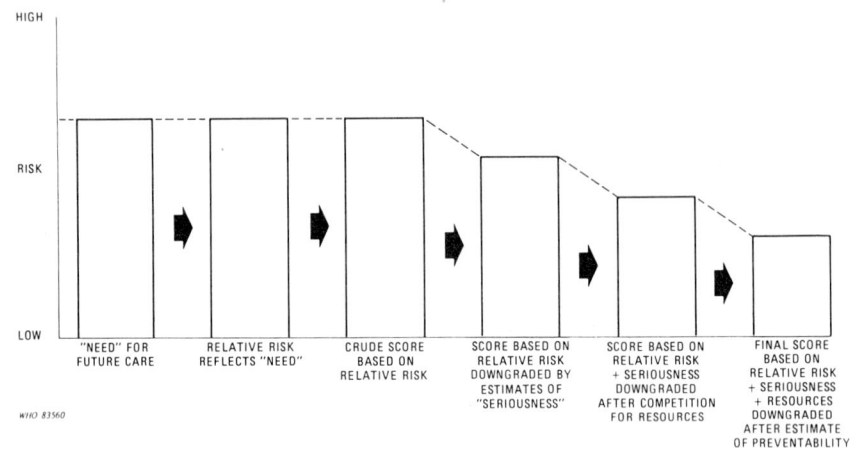

Fig. 8. Scoring and risk: the modification of scores by local values and priorities
(Variations perceived in seriousness, preventability and available resources)

Fig. 8 illustrates this latter approach by showing how a score which at first truly reflected relative risk is modified "downwards" by diminished community concern and resources.

If scoring is used at all (and it is particularly useful in improving referral), it is probably best not to modify scores but to treat them as if they were shorthand indications of need made prior to the decisions as to what subsequent detailed actions must be taken.

4.1.2 Cut-off points and risk

Dichotomous risk factors, such as the presence or absence of a history of perinatal death, present little difficulty in the calculation of relative risk. Continuous variables, on the other hand, have either to be dichotomized or to be subjected to complex mathematical treatment which uses all the data. Two often opposing considerations must apply. First, there is *yield* in terms of the relative risk and prevalence. Clearly a cut-off point, such as the age below which it will be deemed illegal to ride a motorized bicycle, should yield a figure for the maximum saving of life. (Where statistics are available this can, of course, be calculated directly.) But there are other considerations (in this case political) and a compromise will have to be made—a marginal analysis problem familiar to health economists (24). If the example were taken from reproductive care, the cut-off for maternal age, for example, might result in the referral of far too many mothers for hospital care, thus swamping the resources available.

A compromise between yield and resources is therefore necessary and the two together will dictate cut-off points. Fig. 9 and 10, illustrate how cut-off points can affect yield and resource use.

FROM RISK MEASUREMENT TO INTERVENTION 37

Fig. 9. Screening for risk: cut-off points in a continuous variable

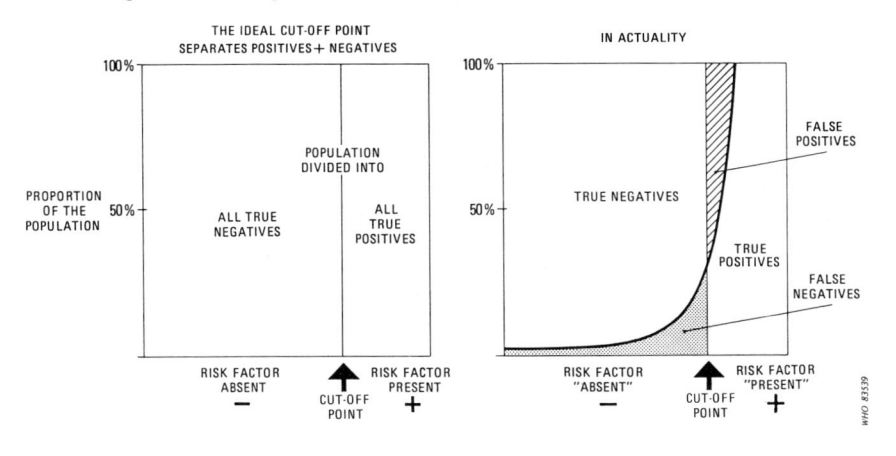

Fig. 10. Screening for risk: "trade-offs" between false positives and false negatives*

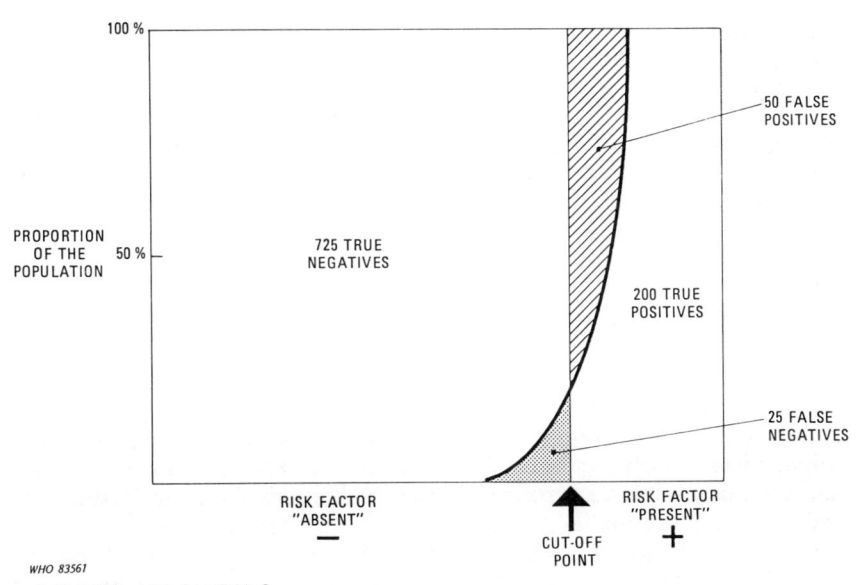

* Hypothetical data from Table 3.

4.1.3 Risk factors and "trade-offs"

While the compromise between yield and resources in deciding the cut-off points of a continuous risk factor is a kind of "trade-off"—the one giving way to the other, but only where absolutely necessary—the "trade-offs" between false positives and false negatives is equally difficult. This balance is illustrated in Fig. 10, which shows in diagrammatic form the figures presented in Table 3 (p. 30).

The conflict that must be resolved is between the 25 false negatives and the 50 false positives who are selected at this particular cut-off point. The question becomes one of how many more false positives can be "afforded" by this community for the desired reduction in the number of false negatives? The answer will depend, of course, on a balance between the seriousness of the false negative mistakes and the damage done to individuals by the needless use of resources on false positives—that is, on people who at first were thought to be at high risk and later were found not to suffer the adverse outcome.

4.2 The Health Care System: How Can it Be Changed?

The community and its services are at this point poised (as it were) on the brink of trying some new uses for all the information about risk. There is, however, one final question (the fourth preparatory step) which must be asked, and that is whether the existing health care system can change sufficiently to accommodate the innovations which will be proposed.

So many variations exist in the organization of health care that it is likely that not all could use the risk approach. Systems without a coordinated referral chain or those run without regional or other coordination are at a particular disadvantage. Plans to use the risk approach would, of course, be fully adapted to local patterns of care, local value systems, local religions and local methods of payment. But such adaptation has limits (for example, financial or operational limits) beyond which accommodation is impossible. Before the innovation is planned it is therefore necessary to describe in some detail the ways in which care is currently delivered (particularly as regards the target outcomes), as well as the existing policies for the promotion and maintenance of health. The main determinants (laws, customs, etc.) of these patterns would also be described, the purpose being at every stage to seek an answer to such questions as: Is the health care system (and its associated laws, customs, etc.) capable of accommodating the risk approach—i.e., can it be changed sufficiently? Or: Is it likely that the addition of the risk approach will help? Are the available health data good enough to make the approach viable? Is there sufficient local, regional and national support for the educational and training programmes involved to give them a reasonable chance of success?—and so on.

4.2.1 The crucial questions

A number of questions will be of crucial importance to the success of the risk approach. For example, while the attitudes of local people and of their government may at first be accommodating, they may subsequently change. Are the people cooperative? Can the local services be organized (with sufficient integrity of the referral chain) to be able to innovate without too much opposition, for example, from private medical care?

The accessibility of records, the possibilities of local reorganization of care, the extent of cooperation of primary and other health care workers, the possibilities of some resource reallocation and retraining, etc., will all need to be evaluated and further scrutiny of the health care system will be required. This assessment will often be difficult but it is prerequisite to a decision as to whether to develop the risk approach strategy, in which situations and to what extent. As will be seen later, there is a large range of possible uses for this strategy so such a decision is rarely a clear "all-or-nothing" choice but rather one which estimates how much of a contribution the risk information can make. Since poorer countries benefit most from any improvement in care, significant compromises will always have to be made, for it is these countries which not only have the greatest need but also the poorest services.

4.2.2 Data for future evaluation and planning

Having made the decision to proceed with the innovation and to try out the risk approach, the accumulated information about the health care system, which has been collected in order to answer the main question—to go ahead or not—assumes a different character. This information now becomes part of an essential set of data to be used in the future as a basis for evaluating the innovation and for planning purposes. If the innovation forms part of routine service improvements, rather than a research project, a smaller and simpler set of data can be the basis of planning. The very least that will be needed are basic vital statistics (or reliable estimates thereof) and a description of the health care and social organization of the community. Some evaluation of services is, however, possible without waiting for very precise information.

4.2.3 Basic information needed for planning the use of the risk approach

Wherever possible the health information for each area should include the following types of data, which, at some stage, may be needed to implement or evaluate the risk approach:[1]

—the age and sex distribution of the population and its geographical distribution by community and household;

—mortality by age and sex and by cause (if possible);

—as much information as is available about local cultural patterns,

---

[1] This list is only an example. It will need modification to suit different areas, cultures, health care systems and uses of risk.

occupations, religious customs, and attitudes to health, disease, and death (in particular the local attitudes to family planning and child rearing would be important);

—information about the services which are likely to experience the most impact from the risk approach—e.g., the referral system, educational facilities and health education services;

—information about environmental risk factors such as deficient sanitation, water supplies, and sewage disposal, and the presence of disease vectors;

—information about local community organization, including women's groups and youth groups, the identity of religious and lay leaders, and local administrative patterns;

—information about how the health problems of mothers and children are at present being dealt with;

—information about local health services, their organization, availability and use;

—information about health care personnel, their distribution by numbers and level of qualification; and

—information about traditional healers and birth attendants and their training, if any.

Not all this information will be available and much will be unsatisfactory in quality. Where the need is vital, it may be necessary to undertake special surveys or make estimates from reports compiled by those with a knowledge of local conditions.

4.2.4 Information needed to establish individual risk

If the risk approach is to be applied to individuals, it will be necessary to make and maintain regular contact with all households in the area to detect risk factors, to monitor outcomes and quantitatively to relate the one to the other.

4.2.5 Information needed to establish community risk

Records indicating the characteristics of neighbourhoods, districts and regions in terms of outcome—the incidence or prevalence of priority health problems—and features such as socioeconomic status, occupation, income level, housing standards, demographic structure, and environmental quality (the related potential risk factors) require information systems unlikely to be found in areas of greatest need. Estimates based on sample studies, or "guesstimates" based on the experience of local people, will probably be all that is available. Vital events and denominators will also probably have to be estimated, as will the derived relative and attributable risks.

A somewhat over-simplified example might be taken from a hypothetical shanty/slum neighbourhood in which some 1000 families could be sampled. In a given year there might be about 3000 children under 3 years of age in this rough sample. From verbal reports there are two sources of water supply, one good and one bad, the good one serving about two-thirds of the population and the bad one the remainder. Fifty-six deaths probably involving diarrhoea and similar illnesses were reported in the last year among the children in the sampled families, 20 of them in the good water area. Among the various factors which might have contributed to these deaths, polluted water is important. How important it is could be estimated as follows: assuming that bad water is a risk factor for gastroenteritis, that the whole community is otherwise homogeneous and that the sample is reasonably representative, the relative risk of the bad water source would be 36 in 1000 children divided by 20 in 2000 children. The relative risk is therefore 3.6—or, very roughly, a 260% excess risk of death associated with the bad water supply.

The attributable risk is the measure needed to support a plea for a better water supply, and that is about 46%, whether calculated from relative risk (the preferred method in this case) or by scrutiny of the probable death rates. This means that if—and only if—this series of "guesstimates" is reasonably accurate, then rather less than half the infant deaths from gastroenteritis could be prevented by extending the good water supply to the one-third of the population lacking it. (It should be noted that even in such crude guesswork as in this example the usual statistical safeguards should be applied, wherever possible.)

4.3 Intervention at Different Levels of Care

The place of information in strategy development has received much attention and there are a number of authoritative works on the subject (see, for example, reference 25). None, however, is especially concerned with the contribution which could be made by data about the distribution and extent of risk in a community. Fig. 11 (p. 43) illustrates some of the ways in which these data might be applied at different levels of care.

The notion of "levels of care" is often used to define the main point of impact of an intervention within the health care system. In the past, the use of risk data has been concentrated on improving one level of *medical* care. Here, scoring systems linked to the relative risk of potentially adverse factors recognized prenatally have been used to improve referral, increase the intensity of surveillance and reallocate resources, as well as, indirectly, to define the medical task.

The risk approach can be applied at all levels of care, from self and home to intersectoral policy. Eight such uses of the risk approach strategy of resource reallocation and care in proportion to need are suggested. Each is put forward because it seems likely to have a positive effect on the health care of mothers and children.

Three of the interventions proposed are outside the formal health care system—the first two at the level of self, family and community care and the third at the most distant level, that of intersectoral policy. Between these three are five suggested uses of the risk approach within the formal health care system (in increasing coverage, in improving referral patterns, in matching health professional skills and individual needs, in the medical attack on risk factors, and in local, regional and national reorganization and training).

For purposes of illustration, these uses of risk data are treated as if they were separate one from another. This would not be the case in actuality, nor would the referral chain be as simple as is suggested. It is also recognized that health care systems, where they exist at all as organized systems, might be a mixture of good and bad care, costly and free care, and sometimes no care at all for those at high risk and too much for the relatively healthy. It is with this kind of real-life system that the risk approach is concerned and in which the applications described in the next chapter seem appropriate.

5. Uses of the risk approach

5.1 Applying the Risk Idea

Experience with the risk approach suggests that the idea of positive discrimination in health care based on measurements of risk is of general value and could be applied to a number of different parts of a health care system. The eight different uses chosen as examples (Fig. 11) are therefore suggestions which, though prompted by experience, constitute a series of hypotheses still to be tested under field conditions. In ideal circumstances a health systems research programme should evaluate each use of the approach before service innovation takes place. The proliferation of such activities not only would satisfy the requirement of research support before general application but would create in each

Fig. 11. Some uses of the risk approach inside and outside the formal health care system

		3	4	5	6	7	
		INCREASING COVERAGE	IMPROVING REFERRAL	MODIFYING RISK FACTORS	LOCAL REORGAN-IZATION AND TRAINING	REGIONAL AND NATIONAL REORGAN-IZATION AND TRAINING	
		RISK SCREENING INCREASES COVERAGE	RISK DATA OR SCORES MEAN NEEDS AND SKILLS ARE BETTER MATCHED	TREATING HIGH BLOOD PRESSURE OR DIABETES, FOR EXAMPLE	CHANGING SKILLS AND FACILITIES TO MATCH NEEDS	CHANGING SKILLS AND FACILITIES TO MATCH NEEDS	
1	2	WITHIN THE FORMAL HEALTH CARE SYSTEM					8
SELF AND FAMILY CARE	LOCAL COMMUNITY CARE					INTERSECTORAL POLICY
SCREENING SELF AND FAMILY FOR RISK, FAMILY HEALTH EDUCATION	COMMUNITY DEVELOPMENT, LOCAL CARE					REFLECTS DISTRIBUTION OF NEED AND RISK FACTORS SUCH AS POVERTY, OVER-CROWDING AND MALNUTRITION

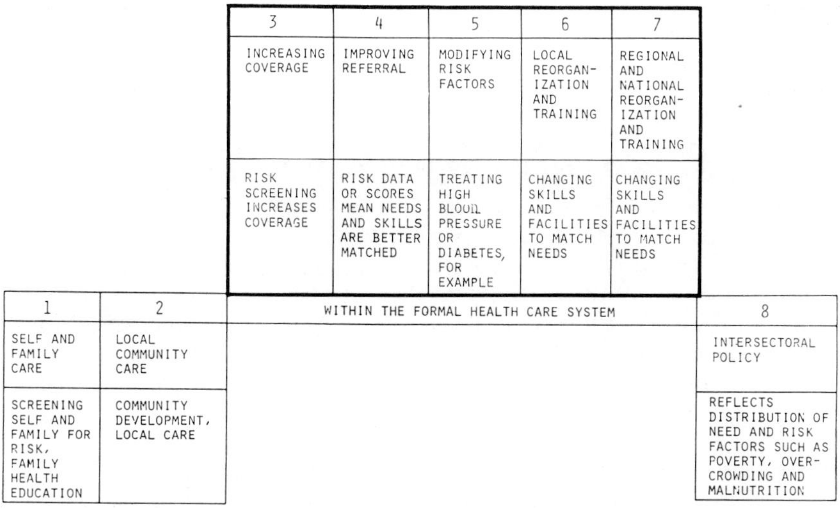

region a cadre of people experienced in health systems inquiries.[1] That this is necessary will be generally agreed but until there are sufficient researchers available some compromise is inevitable. There should still be tests of the effectiveness of the various uses of the risk approach, and continuous evaluation, even of its service uses, is necessary.

While the logic of the risk approach seems theoretically unassailable, this is not enough; it will be necessary to modify health systems research methods and make them appropriate to the testing of hypotheses in real situations. Such methods would simplify evaluation, and the associated sampling, record-keeping, calculating, surveying and data analysis would become more adapted to local skills and resources. An example would be preprogrammed, portable, computerized record systems, which may shortly provide easily understood and simple bases for local surveys. There is still a great need for research into the most appropriate way to generate the relatively complex data used for innovation in health care, particularly at the local level in poor countries, where the task often falls on already overworked village health workers. Moreover, a strong case can be made for integrating all health care programmes at neighbourhood level.

Applications of the risk idea are likely to involve other departures from established health care patterns that reach beyond the need to evaluate. The most important of these is the initiation of contact by the health care system rather than by the patient. To do this successfully requires community participation and a nonauthoritarian approach on the part of officials and health professionals. Because of the traditional mechanisms of care, which respond to those seeking help in times of illness, individual preventive medicine requiring some preliminary screening will be regarded with suspicion for a long time. A response rate of considerably less than 100% must therefore be expected.

Another problem which will be encountered is the need both to provide a curative service and to be seen to provide such a service, particularly during the period when the innovations are being planned and initial screening takes place. Such services are as necessary as a local understanding of objectives.

5.2 Applications outside the Organized System of Care

From Fig. 11 it will be seen that applications of the risk approach are likely to be easier within the organized system of care than outside it—in fact, the ability of that system to accommodate and use risk data is one criterion of acceptability of the approach. However, most health behaviour, most early care of illness and preventive activities of all kinds take place in the home or local community before the individual passes along the referral chain and into the organized system. Because of its importance to the effectiveness of care, this informal system, which, in

---

[1] The necessary training workshops are being held (see footnote[1] on page 15).

fact, is the beginning of the referral chain, has received increasing attention since the introduction of primary health care, particularly from the health educators, from those interested in the family as a social unit, and from such widely differing groups as geneticists and practitioners of folk and traditional medicine. The more that is known of the determinants of maternal and child health, the more important this informal care is seen to be;[1] any improvement in its effectiveness will therefore be rewarding.[2] Two points of possible application of the risk approach are proposed within this informal system of care (see Fig. 11, applications 1 and 2).

5.2.1 Self and family

Strategies which use the risk data at the level of self and family care will depend on the ability to translate and communicate the technical information about risk and the associated need for preventive action in a form which can be understood and does not provoke fear. For this reason a substitute for the word "risk" may have to be found and there may well be existing forms of speech within the family which already accommodate the idea of relative risk with a minimum of anxiety.

Apart from creating a general awareness of what is important and what is unimportant in the maintenance of health, the use of risk data at self and family level might be considered to have three overlapping objectives, as described below.

5.2.1.1 Improved ability to recognize health priorities and health lifestyles and behaviour.

This is the first and most important objective. It implies the adoption of a more rational approach to self and family care, which would replace irrational interpretations of risks. This must not become an assault on existing family values. But the approach could lead, for example, to a better understanding of the benefits of breast-feeding or immunization against tetanus, and of the risk of neglecting these practices, of nutritional care in pregnancy or the early recognition of risk factors for infant gastroenteritis. The establishment of realistic priorities in family health would focus attention on prevention rather than on curative care.

5.2.1.2 Informed surveillance of self and family.

The early recognition of risk factors does not necessarily imply an anxious preoccupation with illness but rather the gradual sophistication of self and family care so that, within the family group, high-risk

---

[1] Health behaviour, the socialization of the child and bonding are, like early risk-taking behaviour, already being established in the young family.

[2] That improvements are called for is suggested by the continuing high morbidity and mortality rates experienced by young families in developing countries.

situations are recognized early and attended to before others of less importance. The family is more alert to threats and potential threats to its health.[1]

5.2.1.3 Earlier self and family referral.
Increasingly informed and responsible health management of the family would involve the early recognition of danger signals, selective referral, and a more critical appraisal of facilities.

The methods which would be used in the application of the risk approach to self and family care are likely to be specific to each culture, but because behaviour does not necessarily change with knowledge alone they would involve much more than didactic explanations of the relationship of risk factors to outcomes. The methods of choice are those of the most advanced and actively involved health educators, the mobilizing of group pressures and integration with community development activities, as well as individual work within the family at times of high receptivity by respected seniors.

5.2.2 The local community

Applications of the risk approach at the local level would seek to spread new information about the nature and extent of the relationships existing between the environment and the health of the individual, the family and the community, and between behaviour and health. Properly interpreted, risk information could become a vehicle for the demonstration of cause and effect in the genesis of disease and help to develop interventions appropriate to the local situation. It would also seek to foster community action in the control of risk factors in accordance with their importance for family and community health. Finally, it would seek to use group and individual risks as starting-points for community action to improve referral and foster an earlier, anticipatory or preventive and promotive approach to primary health care.

The methods which would be used in this application of the risk approach would ensure joint action as well as joint collection and dissemination of information with community development and other local programmes. It would rely heavily on hitherto untapped non-conventional resources—particularly human resources. Village groups, urban neighbourhood groups, "self-help" and women's groups are examples of likely vehicles for the effective spread of new knowledge about the distribution of risk and risk factors in local communities. The most effective way of promoting the use of risk data by the local community for its own care is likely to be through the women of the

---

[1] Recent work in China, details of which were presented at the 1982 Scientific Advisory Group Meeting in Kuala Lumpur by Dr Chen Mei-Pu ("Community involvement in the risk approach", unpublished material from the International Peace Maternity and Child Health Hospital, Shanghai), suggests that routine prenatal screening for risk carried out by the family is highly effective.

village or neighbourhood undertaking the initial screening for risk themselves, with the help of the village health workers, traditional birth attendants and midwives. Shared knowledge of risk at this level offers not only a summary of the state of health of the community, but an indication of which individuals need local and professional help and of the requisite kinds of support, group action and political participation in environmental control.

There is an opportunity here, through social support, to prevent the anxiety mentioned above, to encourage care both outside and inside the health care system and to produce a powerful political and environmental pressure group concerned with promotion of the health of the family in the village or township. Much will depend on what constitute the target health problems of the area, but if, for example, the community has decided that neonatal tetanus and infantile gastroenteritis are high on its list of priorities, so much is known about the risk factors associated with these conditions that a coherent attack should be possible. This would be done by mobilizing local social pressures in order to achieve appropriate preventive action, including improvements in the local environment.

Risk information, appropriately translated, will add force to these arguments by indicating the extent of the problem and by defining which groups and individuals are at different levels of risk. It could also guide the local village leaders (as well as regional and other health managers) towards the most effective community action and towards regional and perhaps national action in the control of risk factors.

In summary, two possible contributions of the risk approach could be developed, one at village or community level and one at family level. They would both exploit the new information about vulnerability, risk and risk factors and thus supplement existing health information. The ways in which this might be accomplished include the use of participant techniques for the transfer of information and the promotion of behavioural change. These methods would respect local value systems and would not necessarily rely on what has been called the "medical model" but work also within any alternative and traditional system of care. Using current patterns of behaviour, they would seek to inform the people about differences existing in the health and potentiality for illness of mothers and children in the local population so that the population itself could assume a greater and better informed responsibility for its own care.

5.3 Applications within the Organized System of Care

5.3.1 Introduction

The risk approach has been the subject of research mainly at the local level, where referral systems, scoring and medical interventions to modify risk factors are, in maternal and child health at least, reasonably well known and where local resources can usually be reallocated.

However, as consideration of how the risk approach might be used passes from the activities of individuals in their homes and village clinics to possible use in the reorganization of health services, the issues become more complex. The information needed changes from familiar medical records and relative risks to costs, benefits, attributable risks and political concerns. Little is known about the part played by such information in determining social policies, and though the health economists are making speedy advances (24), it is probably still small.

The measures which are the tools of the risk approach may therefore have a wider application, though this cannot be certain. If they can be thus applied, they will be particularly useful in national resource allocation—where risk could be used as a proxy for health needs and thus contribute to fiscal policy priorities.[1]

5.3.2 Increasing coverage

The value of the risk approach in increasing coverage is treated separately in this review of possible uses, because, in all the literature on primary health care, improvement in coverage—that is, increasing the number of persons who receive care *of any kind*—is rightly given great prominence: health for all requires access to health care for all.

Of all the factors influencing coverage, three have received particular attention and all may be affected by the risk approach. Availability, access and what has been called "threshold" and acceptability are important determinants of both formal and informal care.

Increasing the *availability* of appropriate care is an objective of the risk approach which, in theory at least, offers a method for reallocating resources according to need, and thus should increase coverage. The procedure involved is a transfer of resources formerly expended on those at low risk to those in greater need—among whom would be some individuals who hitherto have received no formal or informal health care. In reality, it is doubtful if this reallocation could immediately take place so as to reflect the need and increase coverage; when it does, it is likely to be the most effective in clinics and hospitals—that is, further along the referral chain. The screening of the population for risk and the care of those found to be in need of it would, initially at least, use *more* resources—particularly community resources newly mobilized—the overall availability of care being considerably increased. Later, when the principle was understood and applied, the allocation of new resources would be gradually increased according to need. (Most services, except those far along the referral chain, will be effectively bypassed by the privileged few. It is essential to recognize this "second system" of care in all innovations.)

---

[1] The Resource Allocation Working Party for England and Wales uses the Standardized Mortality Ratio as one expression of health needs in the allocation of a small proportion of regional funds within the British National Health Service. Risk data might be more appropriate.

Improvement in *access* to care would take place for the same reasons as increase in availability, and also because the risk approach seeks out those at risk rather than waiting for them to apply to the services for help. It does not follow, however, that improvements in physical access, such as better transport, can be provided without extra resources. The possibility of such improved access—so that mothers and children can be screened and subsequently cared for at the appropriate level of care— is one of the criteria of feasibility of the risk approach. It is to be hoped that sufficient resources will eventually be saved by increased efficiency within the system for the additional costs to be absorbed. However, in practice this is difficult in the context of the efficiency of health care and thus cannot be taken for granted.

The notions of *"threshold"* and *acceptability* as factors in the health care coverage of a population consist in, first, the recognition of personal illness, and then the acceptability of care. Persons with an understanding of the risk factors in family health will respond earlier and more readily, recognizing the need for care (formal, informal and self care) when appropriate. They have a "low threshold", so to speak, and will probably seek health care when it is needed. For some families, however, the threshold is high and the need for health care is not recognized. The reasons for this lack of recognition of need are poorly understood and are, of course, difficult to separate from a reluctance to use services.

A proper use of risk information should lower the threshold and make health care (including self care) more acceptable. It would do this by helping people to understand the nature and extent of the risks and the risk factors involved. It would affect only one part of the barrier between the recognition of need and the seeking of care, the lowering of which is also dependent on a complex of attitudes in which acceptability and the expected effectiveness of care play a large part. It must be remembered that much health care is still ineffective and some aspects of it, particularly the uncontrolled use of powerful drugs, are dangerous. For these reasons risk information might well make some people apprehensive.

Where the assessment of risk and the definition of risk factors are not an individual matter (defining, for example, the risks facing the population using motorized bicycles, or the population of infants with an inadequate water supply or with illiterate parents) then the risk approach does not directly increase health care coverage, although it may well lead to an increase or an improvement in services. Where the individual is concerned, it is expected that it will lead to better coverage. As indicated above, the most important feature of the risk approach which prompts this improved coverage is that contact is initiated by the community and its health care system and not left entirely to the individual. This fact alone is likely to alter the pattern of, for example, prenatal and infant care. Moreover, the effect on community health of such an increase in coverage could well be a disproportionate improvement. This is because there is a marked excess of high-risk persons always to be found among those who hitherto have not elected to seek care at all. For the first time some, at least, of this hidden need will be met.

The resources required for this initial screening are, first, a cadre of moderately trained local people—health workers or traditional birth attendants—an elementary recording system, questionnaires, etc., and, most important of all, a minimum of community organization and cooperation and some primary care for those in need. There must also be local knowledge of the distribution of houses, farms and villages in the area and some means of transport. The screening, whether "research" or "service", should always be combined with care of some kind, and clear decision pathways should be available which will define the frequency of the subsequent contact and the actions to be taken when previously chosen risk factors have been identified. The principle of "no research without service" should invariably be followed.

5.3.3 Improving referral

Improving referral implies facilitating the movement of individuals along the referral chain in order to ensure that all people reach the level and kind of care which they need. It is to be hoped that, at the same time, greater coverage will have been achieved so that more of the people's needs are met by community and health service skills appropriate to dealing with them.

This application of the risk approach, in association with the modification of risk factors, is the one which has had the longest use and which is supported by the most experience. The objective is to achieve the best possible congruence between needs and the facilities and skills available to meet these needs. In reality the use of risk data in this way would never be isolated (as it is now for descriptive purposes) but would be linked with the examples which follow, so that skills, the capacity of institutions, facilities and technologies are enhanced and improved at the same time as referral for promotive and preventive care is made more effective. At this point in the development of these ideas the first objective is to achieve the "best fit" in the existing referral chain without altering the chain itself, thus ensuring that people are referred to the best available skills, facilities, etc., according to their needs. Consideration will be given below (see section 5.3.5) to the possible uses of the risk approach in the improvement of those skills, facilities, etc.

If the risk data are to be used in improving referral there must be a link with the health care system (for example, to facilitate management decisions). A score based on the relative risk is often used for this purpose and is an effective, if crude, indicator of the urgency and seriousness of individual need. Such a risk score is, like the relative risk itself, only a proxy for need; it will subsequently be necessary to examine in detail the nature of the need, the risk factors involved and the facilities and skills, etc., that are available and needed. In this way the object of this part of the risk strategy—a matching of need and skill, etc.—may eventually be achieved. In such a system, mothers with the same risk of a defined outcome will be referred to the same level of institution with the same facilities, technologies and skills. This does not mean that all their needs will be identical but they will fall within the same broad group and, ideally, the institution or clinic of referral will have the capacity, skills and technology necessary to meet them. The use of scores in referral can be illustrated by diagrams of a hypothetical referral system (Fig. 12–14). Fig. 12 shows a possible distribution of

Fig. 12. Linking the distribution of risk, risk scores and the ideal distribution of facilities and skills

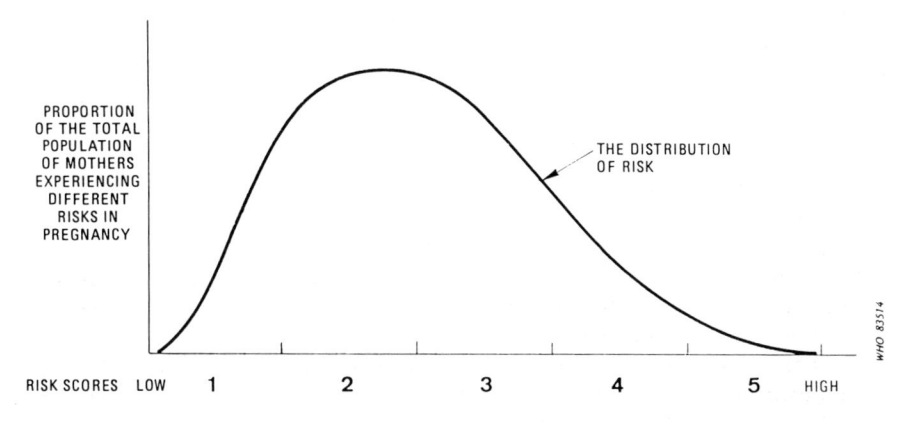

Fig. 13. The ideal referral pattern: a matched distribution of risk and the capacity, skills, etc., of the facility

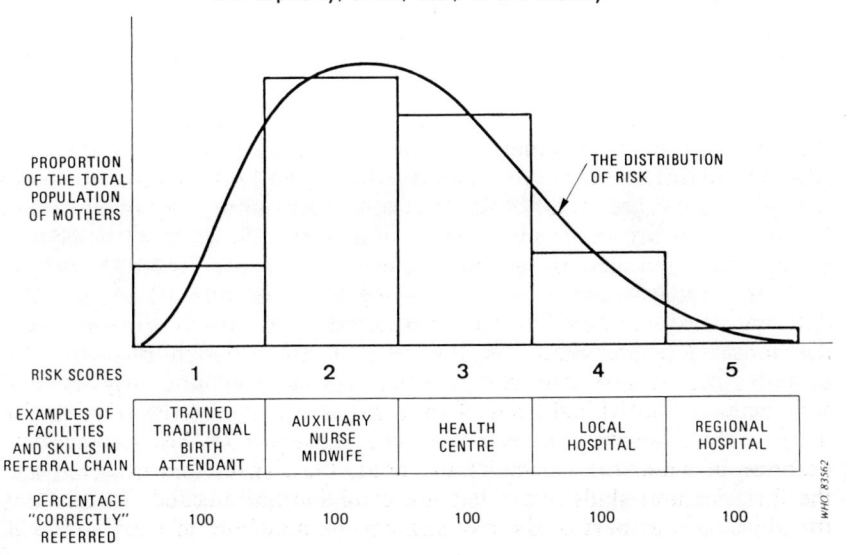

Fig. 14. The referral pattern in actuality: an inappropriate distribution of mothers along the referral chain and, probably, some gross mismatching (hypothetical example)

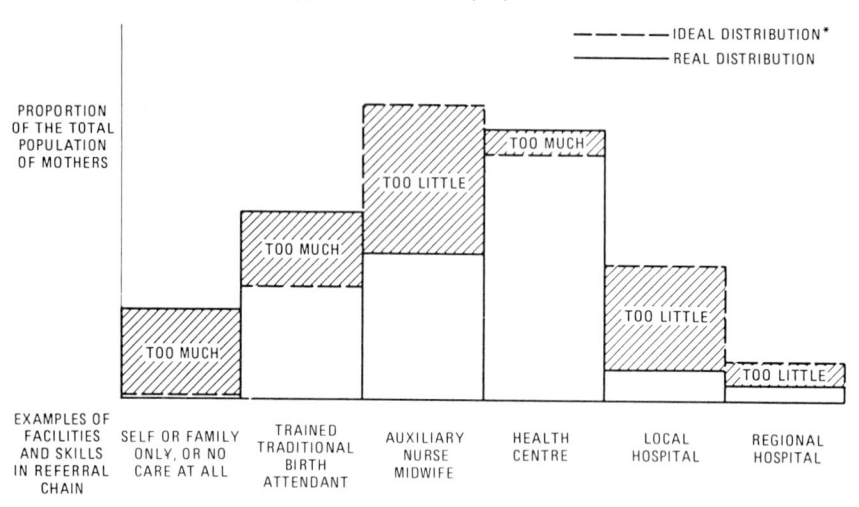

The ideal distribution is where needs for care meet appropriate resources (see Fig. 13 and Table 4).

risks in the population grouped on a simple scale of risk scores 1–5. Fig. 13 shows the "ideal" referral pattern towards which it is the intention to move. In the ideal system there is a congruence of need, facilities, technology, skills and capacity. To achieve this, two kinds of adjustment are necessary: improved referral and improved distribution of skills, etc. This section is only concerned with the former and it is suggested that the risk approach, with the use of the shorthand of scoring, might assist in the "correct" (or the best available under the imperfect circumstances) referral of mothers and children. Fig. 14 shows what probably happens in most referral chains—an inappropriate distribution. There are three features of this inappropriate distribution. First, the number of available places at each level—that is, the capacity—is wrong; secondly, skills, facilities and technology are sometimes under- and sometimes over-used; thirdly, and much more important, the referral pattern is wrong—that is, there is an almost (but not quite) random mix of patients, so that some of those who need advanced care are to be found at a low point on the referral chain or receive no care at all, while low-risk mothers and children are sometimes cared for in hospital.

With the use of a scoring system based on a grouping of relative risks into 5 categories, the "best fit" of needs to skills would mean that no one who scored 5 would receive care at a level below that of the regional hospital, and no one who scored 1 would be cared for above the level of the traditional birth attendant's clinic, and so on along the chain. Table 4 shows how some improvement in the direction of this hypothetical

Table 4. Improving the referral of mothers for preventive care: a hypothetical example

Step	Related risk score	Self or family care only, or no care at all	Trained traditional birth attendant	Auxiliary nurse midwife	Health centre	Local hospital	Regional hospital
		1	2	3	4	5
1	"Correct" percentage of mothers at each level (hypothetical)	0	14	36	30	16	4
2	Percentage of mothers at each level *before* scoring	12	25	20	37	4	2
3	Percentage of mothers at each level *after* scoring	5	19	33	35	5	3
4	Apparent "improvement"	7 out of 12	6 out of 11	13 out of 16	2 out of 7	1 out of 12	1 out of 2
5	Action still needed	Reduce still further	Reduce still further	Increase a little	Reduce a little	Increase	Increase
	Comment	Some improvement, but often those at very high risk accumulate at this level, eventually becoming dire emergencies.	The excess suggests that mothers at higher risk are being treated at too low a level on the referral chain.	Nearly right. The improvement suggests some easing of the traditional birth attendants' workload, but auxiliary nurse midwives are still unpopular.	Still too many.	Still too few. Deficiencies here suggest a continuing reluctance to attend hospitals by those who need the skills, technologies, etc., available therein. The local hospital seems particularly unpopular, and one should ask why this is so.	Nearly right, but are they all scoring 5?

Notes: 1. An advance towards the "correct" proportions at each level suggests only a better congruence of need (as expressed in risk scores) and capacity, skills, etc.—i.e., a better match. However, it would also be necessary to find out if the right people were getting to the right levels. Finally, a comparison of mothers' problems and available skills, facilities, etc., might show discrepancies, which would prompt improved training and redistribution.
2. There is no implication that the higher levels of the referral chain are "better"—merely that more skills, greater capacity, etc., are available.

distribution could be achieved with the use of a scoring system. If this were the result the risk approach could be said to have achieved three of its objectives:

(1) A larger proportion of mothers would be correctly placed—i.e., needs more nearly fit available capacity, skills, technology and facilities.

(2) Most mothers would go to the place where their needs could best be met and fewer of them would receive too low a level of care.

(3) Almost no extra resources would have been used (that is, beyond those expended on the original screening necessary for scoring).

Two other measures are important. The first is the proportion of people who are too low on the referral chain. These are people who are either not given a high enough risk score—they are called *false negatives*—or, for some other reason (such as a well-founded fear of hospitals), do not get as far along the referral chain as they should. Whatever the cause of their appearance at too low a level of care the effect is obviously serious. The other measure is the proportion of people who, for some reason, appear too high on the referral chain. Among these will be some who have been given too high a score; they are called *false positives*. The remainder usually appear too high on the referral chain because, for example, they live near a clinic or hospital or are in some way privileged. Whatever the reason, these people represent a waste of resources or, worse, cause the exclusion of someone having a higher priority for care. The two kinds of error—false positives and false negatives—which arise from the scoring are illustrated in Fig. 9 (p. 37). In the hypothetical example shown in Table 4 we do not know the extent of these mismatches of need and resources, but after the scoring procedure has been applied they are likely to be fewer than before. If among those who still arrive at the wrong destination after scoring there are large numbers who are too low on the referral chain (made up of false negatives as well as others who may be frightened to go higher to the correct level of care) urgent action is necessary, for this is the most serious error in referral.

5.3.4 Modifying risk factors

Intervention in the causes of illness by means of vaccination, health education, treatment of intercurrent illness in pregnancy, or family planning have always been among the classic preventive approaches in maternal and child health. Risk data add to the value of these interventions by giving a priority to risk factors at the individual level, and by making possible the calculation of an attributable risk, which suggests how the community would benefit if the risk factors were removed.

Examples abound of risk factors which can be locally and directly modified. They include infected water, certain kinds of malnutrition, marasmus, dehydration and other precursors of severe disease, and, of course, high parity, short birth interval and pregnancy at the extremes of reproductive life. Health workers can be trained to monitor and to intervene in such pregnancy risk factors as diabetes, hypertension, anaemia and some renal disease. In the developed world long-term cohort studies have concentrated on early risk factors for psychosocial breakdown in childhood and adolescence and for inadequate intellectual attainment and reading ability. The Headstart programmes in the USA had as one of their objectives the modification of some of the more accessible risk factors causing scholastic failure. While most of this work is compensatory and seeks to make amends for high risk, some of it endeavours more directly to modify the risk factors of verbal and other types of deprivation thought to be the root cause of the adverse outcome. By analogy with these programmes, the risk approach should aim to modify the risk factors and, where this is not possible, to compensate for them.

An important part of this attack on risk factors involves training lay members of the community, village health workers, traditional birth attendants and others to recognize risk factors for a variety of unwanted outcomes, to understand the scoring or similar system of grouping relative risks (perhaps with the aid of simple algorithms held by neighbourhood or village health workers) and to modify the risk factors which are the most important and within their competence. Community pressure for the modification of such universal risk factors as a deficient and polluted water supply or the absence of nearby health facilities might also receive support from a recognition of the relative and attributable risks of disease and death associated with them. These community risk factors are similar in their way to the risk factors of, say, high parity, hypertension or diabetes in pregnancy, but with the difference that action at provincial or regional level is necessary. The risk approach therefore very often involves risk factor control at community as well as individual level. (The modification of risk factors is also mentioned in sections 5.3.6 and 5.3.7.)

5.3.5 Local reorganization and training

The use of risk data to assist in the local reorganization of health care and as a basis for the local retraining of health workers is suggested by the "poor fit" of needs with skills, facilities, technology and the capacity of institutions in the referral chain, even after the best possible use of risk scoring (see Table 4, p. 53). Thus, even when a "good" distribution of mothers and children has been achieved (in terms of their needs for care), this will still only be the best available under the less than perfect circumstances. The match of needs, skills, capacity, technology and facilities will still fall short of the ideal. Deficiencies of several kinds will be shown up in the local health care system and will emerge when discrepancies are analysed.

First, there will be "misfits" in terms of the capacity of clinics, hospitals, etc., which have the relevant skills to assist those in particular risk categories, and there will probably also be problems of access and transport.

Next, even when capacity, access and transport problems have been solved (perhaps in part by the redistribution of health professionals) there is likely to be a series of "misfits" in terms of the skills, technology, knowledge, attitudes and even policies needed in different places.

Problems of capacity will not be solved by the risk approach—or any other approach—but guidance as to the direction in which personnel should be moved and the ways in which capacity and facilities should be changed to be more nearly congruent with need will be forthcoming from a knowledge of the distribution of risk in the area. Moreover, savings in one part of the referral chain can be used elsewhere. Even when the "best possible fit" of risk distribution, capacity, facilities and staff has been obtained (perhaps by modest rebuilding, redistributing staff and better transport) there will still be discrepancies, particularly in skills. Task analyses for staff at different levels of care in relation to risk and to the actual health problems encountered will help to define the pattern of training and retraining that is necessary.

Experience gained from the effort to bring down maternal mortality suggests that small groups of mothers with well-known and readily recognizable risks (low or high reproductive age, high parity, poor obstetric history, etc.) are not always correctly placed in the referral chain to ensure appropriate emergency care. There might be, however, a final mismatch of needs and skills, with serious consequences. A review of the tasks involved in the referral sequence reveals three possibilities of failure. Either the early screening and scoring have been defective, or the administrative process of subsequent referral has broken down (perhaps because the mother did not wish to attend hospital), or the skills available at the final referral destination were not adequate. The correct performance of these tasks can become the basis of a modest retraining programme once the frequency and nature of the problem are known.

5.3.6 Applications at regional and national levels

The value of risk information in regional and national planning must depend on how well it can supplement data from other, more routine, sources. These are usually vital statistical data, institutional and service data, and data about the use of health care. It is unlikely that such information will be adequate. However, additional sample population data of some kind can probably be obtained and there may also be some census material from which denominators for vital rates can be derived.

The risk data that are likely to contribute to regional and national planning have been suggested in Table 2 (p. 16). They are:

—The prevalence and incidence of morbidity, the mortality, and other indices of various adverse outcomes in maternal and child health.

—The absolute risk of the various outcomes relative to the total population.

—The risk factors associated with the various outcomes:

(*a*) their *prevalence, incidence and trends in time*;

(*b*) their *predictive power*, the proportions of false positives and false negatives involved;

(*c*) the *relative risks* of different outcomes and combinations of outcomes (these may be associated with the risk factors—alone or in combination; of particular importance are the relative risks for whole population groups sharing risk factors of an environmental, nutritional, socioeconomic, health care and family planning nature); and

(*d*) their *attributable risks*. (For a review of some of the policy implications, see reference 26.)

These risk data are most likely to be of use in the following procedures:

(1) The definition of priorities for action to improve maternal and child health. Priorities would be in terms of breaking the causal pathways between risk factors and ill health and would include social policy action, the design of services, fiscal policy and health systems research—all in conjunction with other regional and national policies.

(2) The provision and siting of institutions (hospitals, clinics, etc.) and the appropriate technology of the referral chain.

(3) Deciding the capacity and staffing levels of institutions.

(4) The definition of educational objectives for all health professionals. Curricular planning based on task analyses defined by risk factors and outcomes. The recruitment, training and deployment of personnel.

(5) The further design of the referral chain and its associated communication, information and transport systems.

(6) Assisting resource allocation (of all kinds) according to need as reflected in relative risks or risk scores.

(7) The provision of data (indicators) for the continuous evaluation of the health care provided.

A major task of regional and national planning authorities is policy development and strategic planning. An example of how risk data might add information of use in planning an attack on, say, perinatal mortality and in the promotion of family planning in a region is illustrated in

Table 2 (p. 16), from which the following information emerges:

(1) The overall perinatal mortality was 26.9 per 1000 births. This figure was probably compared with data from other regions and populations and a crude order of magnitude was constructed. The relative position of this region would then contribute to determining the degree of priority to be assigned to a reduction in perinatal mortality.

(2) In the early 1970s the risk factor of a parity of 4 or more was very common—that is, it was present in about 1 in 5 births. This fact in itself, like the original figure of 26.9 deaths per 1000, indicated to the planners the size of the high parity problem. Likewise, the only slightly less serious social risk factor of pregnancy in a single woman was present in nearly 36% of mothers.

(3) High parity (so defined) carried, in this population, an excess risk of perinatal death of 69%; in the case of pregnancy in a single mother the excess risk was 39%. These are appreciable excesses (though, when compared with others, not dramatic) and show that the strength of the associations was enough to warrant concern and preventive action.

(4) An analysis of perinatal deaths[1] associated with the risk factor of high parity and that of pregnancy in single women (which contributed to the respective increased perinatal death rates of 40.4 and 32.8 per 1000 births) drew attention to antepartum deaths as more important than the other cause groups—congenital anomaly, immaturity, obstetric causes. (The pinpointing of these causes of death probably served to indicate some of the clinical tasks and specific skills involved at different levels in the care of pregnant women and thus provided a basis for an education programme for health professionals.)

(5) The attributable risk of high parity was 11% and that of pregnancies in single women 12%. These figures suggest that a family planning programme which limited the number of children to no more than 3, along with special attention to pregnant single women, would have reduced perinatal mortality by at most nearly one-quarter[2]—say, to 21 per 1000. Since high parity and pregnancy in single women may well be associated with a number of other risk factors, the potential reduction of 23% in perinatal mortality is somewhat speculative. However, these attributable risks undoubtedly sharply increased the priority accorded to family planning in national policies, and they certainly focused attention on the detection and care of the pregnant single woman. A successful attack on all the 4 risk factors enumerated in the table might have yielded as much as a 26% reduction in perinatal deaths.

---

[1] Overlapping risks to mother and child often confuse the issue. The causes of a perinatal death which refer only to the child are only half the story.

[2] As it happens, a very substantial advance has in fact been made in the country concerned since the original data of Table 2 were published.

5.3.7 Intersectoral collaboration

Because of the independent ways in which the executive arms—usually ministries—of countries function, the collaboration of one sector with another in joint enterprises related to health is not common. For example, the health ministry seldom collaborates with, say, agriculture in order to increase the production of a specific item of food and thus promote health. Transport and telecommunications, which also play a role in the health services are, like education for literacy, rarely thought of as assisting in health promotion, particularly of the young family. Yet in each of these examples the intersectoral effects on health are massive. They suggest that more information about the extent of these effects should be of interest to the ministries concerned and that they might even stimulate collaboration by showing the effect of one on the other. The sharing and joint exploitation of risk data by different ministries, even if they did not immediately serve these ends, should be a prerequisite of collaboration. The use of risk data by a number of ministries (at national level) or executive branches of government (at regional level) provides opportunities for collaboration which have not hitherto been available. The data offered must, however, promote this collaboration—i.e., they must show clearly to ministries of agriculture or transport, for example, the beneficial effects of the actions of these governmental bodies on the health of mothers and children. Meanwhile the complex politics of collaboration must not be forgotten.

Intersectoral collaboration in, say, the reduction of maternal mortality or of childhood deaths from accidents will lean heavily on the vital statistics available, as well as on the risk data involved. In each example, risk data will provide further explanations of the processes concerned and will illuminate causes by descriptions of risk factors and measures of relative risks. Attributable risks may serve collaborative social policy development by indicating the likely effects on maternal mortality of, for example, an increase in literacy, the provision of transport, or a reduction in nutritional anaemia. Risk factor analysis of maternal malnutrition might thus lead to a revision of agricultural priorities. For childhood deaths from accidents, the contributions of large families, crowding, poverty, lack of play facilities and inadequate transport regulations could be given numerical weights on which to base choices in policy development.

6. Selecting interventions

6.1 The Potential for Change in Health Care

It will be necessary to attempt an assessment of the potential for change in the health care system prior to any decision as to which, if any, of the applications of the risk approach is feasible. The first steps in innovation in health care have been described in terms of managerial processes (27), but in substance they seek only somewhat more dynamic and detailed answers to the question posed in Chapter 4: How can the health care system be changed? Another review of the data already collected will suggest which, if any, of the applications outlined above is likely to be the best starting-point, what the major constraints are for each of the uses of risk data and where the greatest benefits lie (in terms of the health of mothers and children).

The applications which use risk data in the health education of the family and which seek to improve the effectiveness of self care and mobilize village and community interests, though very difficult to implement, are likely to be the easiest to initiate. Applications of the risk approach which involve changing structures and functions within the health care system will be more difficult. Special interests and status systems may be threatened (for example, private medical practice or the work of established traditional healers), and at the level of regional and national policy there will be other threatened groups as well as substantial political implications of change. Opposition must therefore be expected and if a measure of success could be demonstrated without disturbance, at low cost and backed by enthusiastic local participation it would offer the best opportunity to begin the whole process.

There are three preconditions to the selection of innovations which should be observed. First, an "authoritarian" approach must be avoided. Apart from theoretical objections (which are substantial—see the Declaration of Alma-Ata and its elaborations), the chances of long-term success of innovations in health care in which people have a major role to play in maintaining their own health and which do not achieve full participation appear slim.

The next precondition for intervention in health care using any of the innovations described above is that the innovation should fit in with local concerns. This has already been referred to in a more general context (the selection of unwanted outcomes—see section 3.2) but here it is of more than general importance. The objectives of the innovations being considered must not conflict with local, regional and national policies and priorities, nor with local beliefs, values or religious customs. Usually, however, there is room for compromise and for considerable variation in plans and policies.

A great deal will depend on the third precondition—that of good personal relationships between the local population and the health workers responsible for the innovations (whether they are a research team or a group authorized to introduce changes in services based on previous research). The personal and political blessing of those with responsibility for the programme (be it concerned with services or with research), from the minister of health downwards, must be obtained.

6.2 Criteria for Selection

The establishment of maternal and child health and family planning programmes based on the risk approach requires an estimate of the importance of defined outcomes to the community, of the feasibility of detecting those at risk with local resources and of the acceptability of the intervention. Unless this general information (a prerequisite for the simplest of innovations) is acquired, it will be difficult to introduce the risk approach within the organized system of care. In addition, the following criteria, though not absolute (since some application of the risk approach is probably always possible), will greatly facilitate innovation:

(1) The existence in the area of a health care system the organization of which could accept the risk strategy in one of its applications.

(2) The completion of relevant and satisfactory studies suggesting that the risk approach is likely to be a successful basis for service innovation in the area.

(3) A planning or management team capable of making the innovations—that is, one possessing the necessary management skills and insights.

(4) Sufficient administrative authority within the health care system to make the innovations.

(5) The ability to collect and organize the minimum data necessary for innovation.

It should be noted that the risk approach can probably be applied even where no health care system exists, but with respect to the uses of the approach described in Chapter 5, satisfaction of the above criteria would represent the minimum necessary for success.

6.3 Local Priorities for Action

Local priorities are rarely the same as regional or national priorities. Curative care has greater urgency, and prevention must be expected to have a lower priority even when the causal relationships involved can be seen and understood. There is likely to be some local agreement about unwanted outcomes and the community's priority concerns will probably include the following: maternal mortality, illnesses causing infant or toddler deaths, perinatal mortality, adolescent pregnancy, or adverse outcomes such as deaths from malaria, from motor-vehicle accidents or from gastroenteritis.

Local preferences among possible innovations will be much influenced by the chosen priority targets. Thus, for example, if the objective were to lower maternal mortality, *all* the local population groups would be involved in the innovations, which would probably affect self, family and community care, improve referral and coverage, and result in some retraining of health workers and the reorganization of local services. None of the innovations could be developed satisfactorily without local support, particularly from women's groups, and full local participation in decision-making is therefore essential.

Three difficulties attend the interpretation of local decisions. First, chosen targets may be too vague for the application of the numerical part of the risk approach. For example, "Our priority target is a reduction in all illnesses of children", or "Our priority target is good medical care" may well express local feelings but such aims are not amenable to risk strategy intervention without further analysis. Local priorities should be specific and clearly defined if the relationship between risk factors and outcomes is to be effectively exploited.

Next, chosen innovations may be unscientific and, for example, involve the institutionalization of occult practices. Since most applications of the risk approach would be unsuccessful without local cooperation and respect for local decisions, the team charged with the improvement of health care should discuss, compromise, and seek to reconcile innovations with local belief systems. (In some instances they may already be reconciled—though informally; see reference *28*.)

Finally, the chosen innovation may be distorted because of financial, status, class, caste or ethnic privileges which upset its basis in equity and reverse its principle of favouring the needy. This handicap is, to some extent, universal and more difficult to overcome than other hindrances. A fairly constructed system which maximizes care for those in need would, of course, recognize some classes and castes, as well as poverty, ethnicity, etc., as risk factors in their own right and thus go some way to compensate for undue privilege.

6.4 Local Resources

The main resources to be considered are the following:

(1) *People*, both trained and trainable. Vast potential human

resources, usually untapped, will include those outside the formal health care system who may be mobilized, such as traditional healers, indigenous or locally accepted leaders, women and youth volunteers, teachers, agricultural extension workers and schoolchildren.

(2) *Institutions, facilities and technology.* Apart from buildings and medical equipment, these include supplies of all kinds, transport and auxiliary services. Simple equipment—e.g., for weighing babies or for health education—can often be improvised with local ingenuity to meet local needs.

(3) *Managerial skills.* The ability of a manager or an administrator to organize services and supplies, including the supervision of personnel, the maintenance of discipline, and the ensuring of referral, is essential.

(4) *Health information systems.* At their simplest, these would include a rough census and registration of births and deaths, but they would need to be extended rapidly to include additional items such as a register of pregnant women, complications of delivery, and morbidity in childhood. Attention should be paid to the possibility of linking in a simple way the various records of members of the same family. The goal is a simple information system that would monitor the health of the population, its use of services and the outcome of intervention.

(5) *Funds.* Expenditure need not be substantial, but it will include the cost of training for screening—particularly in the case of the initial screening. Traditional birth attendants or volunteers from the community are perhaps suitable trainees.

The most important local resources are time, commitment, enthusiasm and cooperation, though some managerial skills are also essential. In the decisions which must be made about where the risk strategy should be applied, it is important to separate the acquisition of the tools of the risk approach from their applications. The identification of risk factors and the linking of them to outcomes, the calculation of relative and attributable risk and the accumulation of data on prevalence, incidence, etc., must be considered as a separate, initiating exercise, preferably to be carried out only once every few years in a region or even in an entire country. Guidance from local pilot studies of the various types of innovation will be valuable and it will be necessary to test in this way each of the steps involved.

6.5 National Priorities for Action

Estimates of costs and benefits will, at the national level, be subordinated to political and policy considerations, particularly about priorities for primary health care. The choice of the risk approach, and the extent of its application, will depend mainly on the chances that the strategy will in fact improve the health of women and children, but five other national considerations should be recognized:

(1) Usually some kind of organized maternal and child health and family planning programmes exist, which may command local and national respect and which may already be integrated into primary health care. Innovations not only must have support from data before they can be adopted but must also be capable of being accommodated within these existing programmes.

(2) It will be necessary to convince the major health professional groups of the desirability, feasibility and viability of the proposed changes.

(3) Support must be gained from women's organizations and other pressure groups which influence political decisions regarding health policies, particularly those in the domain of family health.

(4) The status of the health ministry *vis-à-vis* other ministries will influence the possibilities of intersectoral collaboration in the use of risk data. In particular, collaboration with community development programmes (which are often intersectoral) will be of importance.

(5) In countries in which payment for health services is usually on a fee-for-service basis or in which private insurance schemes cover all but the poorest, innovations will have to accommodate and work with these complex systems.

6.6 A Decision Pathway

A logical approach to the selection of interventions based on defined outcomes, risk factors, human and other resources, and constraints should be capable of being presented as a series of steps or decisions. However, so many different approaches are possible that only rough guidelines can be given. This is because of variations in the frequency and importance of different outcomes in different localities, as well as differences in risk factors, the quality of data, and available resources, and therefore in the potential of different interventions.

There are two main pathways for the innovations which are the subject of this book: that of *research* and that of *service*. They overlap, but the testing of the risk approach as a health systems research project from which generalizations can be made and on which future services can be based is different in emphasis from that which is described below, which represents the development of the services themselves. The main steps involved are shown in Fig. 15 and 16.

When it has been decided to introduce innovations in the health care of mothers and children and that the risk approach will be used (Fig. 15, steps 1 and 2), the question then arises whether local cooperation and participation are sufficient to permit such changes. This community support is essential (step 3). Next comes the question of adequate background information about the region or area. Is enough known about the population structure, the health care system and how it functions, etc., to permit the innovations without the need to conduct

Fig. 15. Steps in the preparation of the risk approach

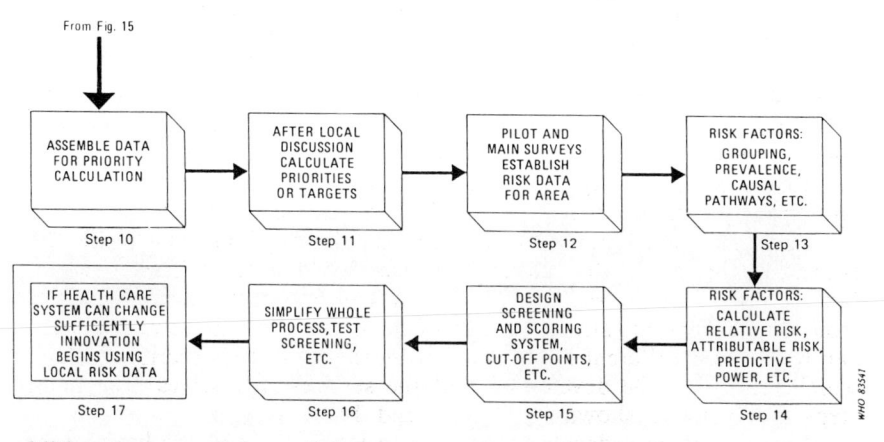

additional surveys? (step 4).[1] From a review of available data it should be possible to decide whether the health care system can be changed sufficiently to initiate the process of innovation (step 5). The same question will have to be asked again when the information about risk

---

[1] Even if such information does not exist there may be reasons for not carrying out surveys—for example, their cost and difficulty—but great care should be taken in design and evaluation if it is decided to omit them.

has been collected; at this stage it would be unwise to proceed unless it seems likely that the risk strategy can be applied. A corollary of step 5 is step 6. Can priorities—the target unwanted outcomes—be defined in sufficient detail to allow the innovations to proceed? In the absence of adequate information, consultations and perhaps small sample surveys will have to be undertaken. Step 7 is a complex series of decisions as to which applications of the risk approach are most needed (in the light of the priorities decided at step 6 and the current effectiveness of the health care system), and step 8 places these decisions within a programme of work (if research rather than service is the objective, this programme would be the "research protocol"). Finally, with these preparatory decisions taken, the collection of information about maternal and child risks in the community can begin (Fig. 16).

Fig. 16 takes this summary of the early part of the process of innovation through 8 more steps, after which the risk data can be used.

Steps 10 and 11: Begin to select the priority targets of the risk strategy from the lists of local health problems; these are the unwanted outcomes. Using the method outlined in Annex 1 decide on their order of priority. The incidence and prevalence of these target outcomes and the concern of the local community will have been ascertained during this process, as will measures of severity, preventability and their trends in time.

Steps 12 and 13: Undertake surveys to establish the risk data for the area. Select the corresponding risk factors. Decide on optimum groupings. Ascertain their incidence and prevalence and describe as far as possible the steps in the causal pathways which link them to the target outcomes. It will be necessary at this stage:

(*a*) To decide whether these causal pathways can be interrupted using available health technology and to determine what the result is likely to be.

(*b*) To decide on the methods needed for measurement (for instance, ascertaining low birth weight requires the use of weighing instruments—which may take the form of a simple balance using stones of known weights, or market-place scales—and someone trained in their use; the diagnosis of fetal anoxia requires even more skill, perhaps a knowledge of how to use Apgar scores, and so on).

(*c*) To determine the feasibility, including the acceptability, of each intervention contemplated in the community in question. This would include a consideration of costs, the use of resources of all kinds, and the size and composition of the populations concerned. It would also include a measure of the resources already available.

Step 14: Calculate the predictive power of the risk factors and their relative and attributable risks.

Steps 15 and 16: Design a screening and a scoring system and test them and cut-off points to see if they are effective. Simplify as far as possible and describe what training has to be given if the plans are to succeed. (Since a certain amount of personnel training will be necessary, the instructions for these procedures would best be summarized in some simple kind of operations manual.) Pay particular attention to the medical interventions and to the accuracy of screening, and keep calculations and the number of risk factors to a minimum.

Step 17: The next step in the service application of the risk approach can be taken when all the necessary information has been collected. Once more the question is asked whether the health care system is capable of accommodating the new strategy. If the answer is that it is indeed capable, and if the local population is supportive and the administrative hierarchy of the region and perhaps of the country is prepared for the changes, then the innovation can begin.

The sequence of innovation could start within or outside the formal referral chain.[1] It should be "run in" until all those involved are "comfortable" with the system—particularly the sensitive processes of screening and scoring. Next, when the system is functioning well, the information could gradually be introduced to improve the referral mechanism. This might be followed by some modest physical reorganization of the institutions in the referral chain, after which the need for some retraining would become obvious.[2] In the meantime, regular meetings with the local people, administrators and headmen would have ensured that what would be a rather slow and modest innovation, at this stage, would be understood and accepted.

---

[1] Any description of how an innovation in health care might come about is in danger of appearing too dogmatic, too optimistic and even paternalistic. Experience of the risk approach applied to scoring and referral suggests that the sequence might be roughly as described.

[2] Some training for screening will already have begun. The aim of the retraining referred to here is to achieve greater compatibility between the needs and skills within the referral chain. For example, it might begin with the training of traditional birth attendants and, at the other end of the referral chain, the training of doctors and nurses in the management of obstetric emergencies.

7. Monitoring and evaluation[1]

7.1 Introduction

In many countries the risk approach will not be applied with full statistical rigour but more often as a guiding principle which, it is hoped, will improve an existing service for maternal and child health including family planning. Therefore, it will not always be subjected to a stringent evaluation in spite of the accepted rule that the value of all health care innovations should be measured. Some improvement in the biological indices—the unwanted outcomes—is likely even without innovation and major ameliorations in care. A more substantial improvement may not be apparent for some considerable time, and even then "proof" of the value of the interventions will not be readily available. It might be possible, however, to demonstrate a reduced frequency of undesired outcomes in defined subgroups of the population, such as fewer obstetric deaths, or a decrease in the number of infant deaths as a result of fewer high-parity pregnancies. Other examples would be a reduction of neonatal tetanus by the immunization of pregnant women or an increase in birth weight through the better recognition of the risk factor of maternal malnutrition.

A number of intermediate or indirect biological outcomes or indicators might also be used (though of necessity with great care)—for example, poor growth instead of frank malnutrition, low birth weight instead of a host of adverse outcomes during the perinatal period, haemorrhage instead of death from haemorrhage, and obstetric emergencies instead of deaths in childbirth.[2]

The incorporation of measures of service use (sometimes called "process indicators") and indirect outcomes as additional indicators of the effectiveness of innovation makes evaluation simpler, though, again, great care must be taken in their interpretation. These process indicators would include, for instance, the proportion of women seen by the health

---

[1] See reference 29.

[2] Absolute figures are often indicative of progress; thus the decline in the number of maternal deaths in a rural region from a steady 8 per year to zero for 2 years running is welcome and suggestive, though probably not statistically significant.

services during their pregnancy, the stage of pregnancy at first contact, the number of contacts for child care, the proportion of mothers immunized against tetanus and of infants completing immunization schedules, and the proportion of women practising family planning. It is reasonable to assume that indicators such as these will, in the long run, reflect the health status of the family and, over time, help to produce the hard data necessary for epidemiological assessment.[1]

Because so much is still unsure about the risk approach, it is particularly important that all its uses should be monitored and evaluated, even if such critical observation is modest, unsystematic and based only on the opinions and feelings of participants.

7.2 Monitoring Health and Health Care

7.2.1 Records

For all evaluation and for the efficient conduct of a health care system, a minimum of three kinds of record must be kept. First, records of the health problems of individuals and families (including their risks) must be collated so as to form a sequential picture of illness and health, of growth and development and of cause and effect over time. Next, these individual records must be brought together to show a *collective* picture of the health of whole populations, also over time. Finally, records of all aspects of care and the outcome of care, including prevention, will complete this minimum description of the community's health.

7.2.2 Skills and insights

In order to answer questions about the health care system and about the value of any innovations in care, five sets of skills and insights are needed: those of the epidemiologists and statisticians, those of the managers and administrators, those of the behavioural scientists, those of the health professionals, and those of the local people—the consumers of care. The ascertainment of accurate denominators and adequate sample size, the design of record systems, the setting of confidence limits, accuracy in coding and tabulating, and the determination of levels of significance demand statistical and epidemiological skills. To work with an indigenous population in a situation of equal participation requires the skills and insights of the behavioural scientists, and innovation in a health care system would not be possible without the assistance of health professionals or managers and administrators. Finally, nothing would be possible without local support and insight.

---

[1] Great care must be exercised in the interpretation of process indicators because more health care does not always means better health care, though in poor countries—particularly those with poor coverage—it often does.

Innovation in health care is therefore becoming increasingly complex as the questions asked—Does it *actually* work? Has the people's health *actually* improved?—become more searching.

7.2.3 Costs and benefits

A major constraint on health care innovation is cost and the principal problem facing innovators is the difficulty of quantifying benefits. To weigh in the balance an innovation, of which the cost is known but the benefits cannot be calculated, means that where money is scarce innovations are rare. In addition, improvements in care are often difficult to demonstrate for so much ineffective care passes as "good".[1] These are some of the difficulties which attend the evaluation of innovations; they are particularly acute where innovation is in health promotion and preventive medicine, and where no dramatic curative high technology is involved. However, one advantage of most of the applications of the risk approach which have been discussed is that they conserve, reallocate and sometimes even "recycle" resources. Because they are, in essence, suggestions as to how to make existing methods of care more effective and efficient, traditional economic cost–benefit analysis should not be the only criterion by which they are evaluated.

7.3 Appropriate Health Systems Research and the Obligation to Inquire

A major paradox facing those who wish to evaluate aspects of primary health care is that many of the commonly used research methods are inappropriate to the context, particularly the context of the village or urban slum, and to the early stages of the referral chain. Attempts have been made to reconcile a dedication to scientific objectivity with the primary health care context of health systems research through the notion of appropriate research. By this is meant such activities as the traditional birth attendant's inquiring whether she is consistent in the numbers of mothers she refers, or the village health worker's finding out whether the dosage of the elementary drugs that he or she is administering is effective. The training involved in such "appropriate" research, or simple inquiry, is more complicated than would at first appear, for it involves not only asking the right questions but a readiness to accept criticism. This objectivity coupled with the obligation imposed on all workers in health care to ask questions critical of themselves and of the system is a suitable training objective and is necessary for any evaluation.

---

[1] There is much to be said, however, for categorizing as "good" that which is accepted as "good", and a basic principle of primary health care is respect for alternative medicine. Moreover, modern medicine is such a powerful weapon that, if it is to be used at all, it must be used properly.

Measurement of the effect of innovations using the risk approach can be undertaken at three levels of sophistication. First, there is the evaluation through lay reporting by the village worker, the traditional birth attendant and the community itself. Next, there is the routine evaluation which should come from service statistics and which should include the use of process indicators and other measures. Finally, there is the more sophisticated health systems research project, in which the statistical rigour and reliability of conclusions will allow of wide generalization. For all three levels of sophistication a study protocol or programme will be of value as a guide to objectivity; for the health systems research project it is a necessity.

7.4 Steps in a Study Protocol

A protocol or programme for a health care evaluation study will contain four main elements. At its simplest it will describe, first, the setting of the problem to be tackled, then the problem itself—the one arising from the other—then what is already known of the subject (the literature review), and, finally, what is to be done to answer the question or to test the hypothesis. This latter section (the main bulk of the protocol) is usually divided into three subsections: that concerned with the methods to be used; the form in which the results will emerge; and, finally, a section on how the conclusions will be drawn from the results. Most health systems research protocols follow this pattern, though, of course, the details will in most cases be more complicated. Under "Method", for example, there will be descriptions of populations, sampling, instruments of survey, data coding and processing, as well as the usual, requisite constraint analysis. An important item will be whether a control population is to be studied in order to provide the investigators with valid comparisons. The protocol will include the form (tabulations) in which results will be presented. Finally, there will be a logistical section on transport, timing, personnel, training manuals, etc.

Under the section on how the conclusions are to be derived will be included lists of the criteria to be used to evaluate the innovation and notes on the size of differences (before/after, case/control, etc.) which will be deemed convincing (significant).

Since all health care should be evaluated, and it is reasonable to refer to all objective inquiries as research, "appropriate" research is that kind of inquiry which fits the context and is compatible with the resources available. For all inquiries involving health service innovations, however simple, the sequence of thinking and planning should follow the ideas expressed in the protocol outlined above. This does not mean that appropriate health systems research is impossible without elaborate statistical methods, but it does mean that it is impossible without some kind of objective appraisal such as that specified in the protocol. Nor is a critical subjective study ruled out, for such qualitative material always supplements and enriches objective population data.

7.5 Evaluation as Part of Health Systems Research

If the evaluation of the risk approach is to be a sophisticated health systems research project, then detailed planning, funding, recruiting of personnel and data collection and analysis will be involved. Research design and protocol preparation will be of great importance, and it should be possible to generalize widely from the results.[1]

In particular, it will be necessary for each research project to include in the protocol operational definitions stating precisely the tasks to be performed at each step, who will perform these tasks, and how and when they will be performed. In short, it will be necessary to write a detailed study protocol that can become the basis for the research. In addition, the research objective will impose certain constraints which would not be necessary for service applications—for example:

(1) It will be possible to select only one or two unwanted outcomes, common, perhaps, to several research centres, in order to permit the comparison of different areas and different uses of the risk data. It is essential if more than one population is under scrutiny that the outcomes selected should be of importance to all areas, although their priority ranking might differ from place to place.

(2) The size of populations to be studied will depend on the strictness of the proposed evaluation and will be influenced by the selected outcomes and their frequency (and, of course, by the time and money available). If, for instance, an attack is to be made on perinatal mortality, of which the initial rate is 40–50 per 1000 births, and the time available is only 1 year, then it would be necessary to obtain, say, 200 cases—i.e., apply the strategy to a population of at least 4500 pregnant women.[2]

(3) The duration of the research should be as short as possible but it will probably take 3 years. This will depend on the frequency of occurrence of the outcome selected, the availability of personnel, the speed of development of the innovation to be evaluated and the quality of the data generated. The steps outlined in Fig. 15 and 16, which must be taken prior to the innovation, are likely to use up an appreciable proportion of the total study time.

(4) Any comparisons between different programmes in different areas will have to use the most rigorous methods. The difficulties of this type of comparison are considerable but may be eased, in part, by standardization and coordination. It should be possible to use designs which can be changed and in which modifications to projects in one area are made on the basis of results from that and other areas. Such a

---

[1] Training programmes for research workers are under way in three WHO regions, and a workbook is available (see footnote[1], page 10, and footnote[1], page 15.)

[2] Sample size is, of course, of critical importance in all population studies.

scheme, properly devised, could be analysed to give rapid and valid results.

(5) The geographical areas of the research should, of course, be chosen by the countries concerned in the light of the existing constraints and local need. Criteria for selecting these research areas should include the following:

—the area should not be too remote or inaccessible;

—minimum data should already be available about the population—e.g., census and vital statistics—or they should be made available without undue difficulty;

—some basic health services should already exist, and there must be a possibility of developing these to permit contact with every woman and child—in other words full coverage must be feasible, even if the primary health worker concerned has had only minimal training;

—the local community should be enthusiastic, wholehearted support should be given by the authorities, and full collaboration should be provided by all health and social services;

—there should be no major bar to the use of services—i.e., most services should be available free or at low cost;

—the political situation should be relatively stable;

—later integration of the innovation into local, regional or even national health plans should be feasible;

—health care resources, even if limited, should be capable of reallocation, and it should be possible to carry the research through with only a few added resources, except, perhaps, for additional training facilities;

—there should be access to comparable areas which could act as control areas.[1]

7.6 Routine Evaluation of a Service Innovation

The routine evaluation of a service innovation that includes the risk approach has been the main theme of this chapter and, though the protocol which should guide this process involves the same sequence of steps as in the testing of the approach as a health systems research project, it is less rigorous. For this reason there is likely to be less certainty about the conclusions; the evaluation is simply part of what should be a regular and obligatory process (for ethical reasons) for the

---

[1] Not only the ethics but the possibility of conducting case-control studies must be carefully and critically considered. The possibility of "experiments of opportunity"—that is, of access to comparable data from what is virtually a control area—must be explored.

monitoring of all innovations—a process which should be going on in all health care systems based on primary health care, if progress toward the ideal of health for all is to be achieved.

7.7 Evaluation Criteria

The objective of all the innovations which use the risk idea is a significant reduction in the unwanted outcomes. The hypothesis on which the evaluation is based can be stated in simple terms such as: "That the use of this innovation will reduce significantly, etc., etc.", and this proposition can then be tested. However, it is not always possible to measure with sufficient accuracy for statistical proof—or the procedure might be too difficult[1] or too costly, or it might take too long. For these reasons it is often necessary to fall back on process indicators of improvement in care, and for reasons already stated these must be interpreted with caution. In spite of these reservations and the care with which a drop in death or illness rates must be interpreted (they may, like heart disease or stomach cancer mortality in developed countries, be declining for different reasons in different places) all relevant criteria must be used—both "outcome" and "process". Thus, for example, the extent of coverage, the knowledge and use of risk data by the community, "improved" referral patterns, more relevant training programmes, and a referral chain more congruent in its skills with the needs of patients can all be used as indicators of "successful" innovation.

As a further illustration of the pitfalls attendant on all evaluation, particular attention must be paid to the previously mentioned Hawthorne effect (see section 3.4.3). This is a positive effect on the unwanted outcome—say, infant gastroenteritis—in a population, which results entirely from the process of being studied and of being the subject of interest, excitement and report, rather than from the interventions of the programme itself. The positive effect of the innovation, to be convincing, must be sustained; it must be plausible, repeatable, and if possible demonstrate some "dose-response" relationship.

In the brief examples which follow, one or two simple criteria are used to show how each of the eight illustrations of possible uses of the risk approach (see Chapter 5, sections 5.2.1–5.3.7) might be evaluated.[2] In addition to these indicators of the effectiveness of the innovation (does it do what it is claimed it will do?), evaluation will also involve an estimate of efficiency (or yield per unit of cost) and acceptability.

---

[1] It is often difficult to relate innovations using different resources to changes in outcome. One proposal is to assign a score to the effect on outcome. Thus, if a given number of prenatal visits (and the interventions consequent on them) reduce perinatal mortality by 10% then these visits score 0.1. Delivery by an obstetrician might lower the perinatal death rate by, say, 8% and so be given the score 0.08, and so on. However, the studies necessary to obtain such data are themselves difficult.

[2] In all evaluation the base-line, or starting-point, is of great importance. Where possible, it should be a clear and unequivocal measurement which is stated in the objectives prior to the innovation.

7.7.1 Application of the risk approach to self and family care

The objectives of this application of the strategy are increased knowledge and use of risk factors within the family. In essence this means that the family knows, in very rough terms, the relative importance of some of the universal risk factors and is using this knowledge in its own care. Proper health behaviour reflecting a knowledge of risk, correct self-referral, earlier attendance for prenatal care by those at higher risk, and so on, would be the kind of indicators which could be measured.

7.7.2 Use of the risk approach by the local community (neighbours and village members)

The objectives of this use of the strategy are much the same as those of the use within the family, though some community action is implied. A first screening carried out by village people, cooperation in training and working with village health workers, more appropriate local referral, earlier prenatal care for higher risk, better coverage and more family planning would be the type of indicators which might be developed for service use. Other indicators of community participation and understanding should be added where possible.

7.7.3 Increasing coverage

All estimations of risk among individuals in a population must increase coverage—at this stage, the notion of the appropriate place for care in the referral chain is not being considered—and increasing cooperation with screening would be a crude but useful measure of success. There will be others—for example, a decline in the proportion of births without a skilled attendant (or births for which risks have not been estimated prior to delivery).

If "coverage" implies that care is available when needed, it would be necessary to ensure that all contact comprises both diagnosis and service, and to monitor to what extent this actually occurs.

7.7.4 Improving referral

Improved referral means that more mothers and children eventually find their way to the point on the referral chain which can offer the best available care for their needs. In the present description, this objective is treated separately. In reality it would be a part of subsequent innovations, which would also seek to improve the distribution of skills, capacity, facilities and technology. If a scoring system based on relative risk is used, the conceptual framework for evaluation has already been indicated (Fig. 12–14 and Table 4). In these simplified diagrams a score is given for each step in the referral chain. This score represents, as far as possible, the competence, skills or ability available at that step and is, under the local circumstances, the most suitable destination for mothers and children having that score. Needs and skills are therefore matched as well as they can be without a radical reorganization of the system. The risk strategy is effective (in this particular application) when *all* mothers and children having a particular score arrive at the appropriate destination (Fig. 13, p. 51). Achievements of this application of the strategy are therefore measured by:

(1) An increase in the number of correct placings—i.e., greater congruence of need and skills, etc.

(2) A reduction in the number of incorrect placings, involving perhaps more than one point on the referral chain.

(3) In particular, a reduction in the number of incorrect placings which are (*a*) at too low a point on the referral chain (i.e., cases that are false negatives and perhaps involve high-risk mothers who have been missed), or (*b*) at too high a point so that skilled workers are used for simple tasks and resources are wasted.

Such an evaluation would depend on record systems which permit the follow-up of individuals to ensure their correct location on the referral chain, provide reliable risk scores, and describe adequately the ability of institutions and health workers.

7.7.5 Modifying risk factors

Individual risk factors which are capable of modification are exemplified by some taboos and cultural practices (though these are particularly resistant to change), malnutrition, poor birth spacing, inadequate family planning, lack of concern for environmental hazards, unsatisfactory personal hygiene, negligent or dangerous work patterns, and numerous intercurrent illnesses. Some can be modified without delay; some will have to await modification till the next pregnancy; while yet others will only be changed in the next generation. An informed attempt at modification is probably the most useful immediate indicator for evaluation, since the effectiveness of such modification is not so easily judged. For a true evaluation, however, real outcome indices must be used.

Modification of community risk factors is probably the most important potential achievement of the risk approach. Once again, the informed attempt at modification as well as the result must be considered.

7.7.6 Local reorganization and training

Improvements in the proportion of correct referrals, though an indicator of achievement of a risk strategy, take no account of the requisite skills, technology, facilities and capacity of institutions within the referral chain. Thus, even if 100 % of mothers and children have been correctly placed with, say, the traditional birth attendant or at a health centre, it may still be that the birth attendant is inadequately trained, that the capacity of the health centre is inadequate, or that the staffing is inappropriate to the tasks involved (see Fig. 16, p. 65). The risk approach in local reorganization and training rests on the prevalence of mothers and children with different needs (and therefore requiring different skills, technology, etc., in their care) and uses that prevalence to guide local reorganization of health care and training programmes. The objective is therefore one step beyond the improvement of referral and consists in modifying the situation so that all features of the referral chain exactly accommodate the distribution of local needs.

A way of measuring progress towards this objective and the relevant conceptual framework were discussed in section 5.3.5.

7.7.7 Regional and national strategies

The value of risk data in strengthening regional and national health services depends on the use made of community risk factors (based on geography, climate, education, occupation, income, food supply, water supply, transport, health care, etc.) and how far they are controlled, the attributable risks (where these can be calculated with confidence) and the nature and prevalence of individual risk factors and unwanted outcomes in the population. These are relatively new data and their use in planning has not been tested to any great extent. Probably their main application would be in decision-making and priority-setting, in cost–benefit analysis and in day-to-day management, though data on attributable risk could help to indicate the risk factors or combinations of risk factors whose modification or elimination would have the greatest effect on the various unwanted outcomes. Risk data could thus become a tool of health and social policy. Prevalence, incidence and time trends could be used as indicators of the size of the task and as starting-points for task analyses and training programmes.

Evaluation of such contributions to planning would be difficult because of the many other factors involved (political, fiscal, etc.), but if specific targets were set some evaluation would be possible. Defined objectives might, for example, specify that:

—20 % of resident doctors at the regional hospitals have (by a certain date) to be capable of undertaking emergency Caesarian section and the hospitals are appropriately equipped;

—all auxiliary nurse-midwives are able to insert intrauterine devices;

—all traditional birth attendants satisfactorily complete 1 month's training within the next 2 years;

—the number of nurse-midwives capable of prenatal and infant screening for risk factors reaches 3 per 1000 pregnancies within 1 year;

—all health workers take every opportunity to encourage mothers to breast-feed their children, so that, within 1 year, the proportion of mothers breast-feeding their children for at least 4 months after birth will reach "X"%.

Evaluation would assess the success or otherwise of such policies.

A rewarding way of tackling such problems as low immunization rates for neonatal tetanus at regional or national level might be to identify population risk factors for "nonresponse", such as service organization deficiencies, religious and cultural prejudices, and illiteracy, thus defining the populations at whom special efforts, policies, or programmes might be directed. A measure of the effectiveness of such an exercise would depend on the accuracy of the priorities later accorded to the control of these community risk factors.

7.7.8 Intersectoral strategies[1]

The use of risk data as a specific stimulus to intersectoral collaboration has been discussed briefly. The contribution of such data is likely to be most clearly seen in the allocation of priorities for health among policies formulated by other ministries in their estimation of the size and nature of the task and the probable effect on the health of mothers and children. The contribution of other sectors to health is more difficult to measure even than that of the health services. In consequence, it is difficult to see how such a multisectoral contribution could be evaluated.

However, where relative and attributable risk for communities sharing certain risk factors can be calculated, subsequent intersectoral allocation of resources (for example, to transport or agriculture) aimed at their reduction would be a good but crude (and indirect) indicator of the effectiveness of this potential use of risk data.

---

[1] The overlap with regional and national strategies—particularly in terms of risk factors—is considerable. Intersectoral strategies are treated separately, since they present a special problem outside the scope of the formal health care system.

8. Lessons from the risk approach

8.1 Application to the Whole Field of Primary Health Care

The underlying idea of the risk approach—that health care and policy should be guided towards prevention by a numerical assessment of future need and should thus discriminate positively—has been widely accepted. What began as a technique for alerting those caring for pregnant women has become a way of thinking about matters as widely disparate as the prevention during childhood of the forerunners of heart disease of middle age, scholastic failure, accidental injury, and adolescent pregnancy. The conceptual framework for a considerable expansion of the risk approach has therefore already been constructed and, although there are special reasons for its usefulness in the case of women and children, there would seem to be few barriers to applying it elsewhere, particularly in primary health care. One reason for caution, however, must be the shortage of support from the results of evaluative research so far, and another lies in the very attractiveness of the idea itself.

The shortage of support from evaluative research is attributable to two factors. First, health systems research in the context of primary health care in developing countries is very difficult to carry out, and, secondly, the studies which are now under way will, of necessity, take a relatively long time to complete, if they are to provide valid results.

However, there is good reason to believe that research support is now forthcoming from these studies.

The attractiveness of the idea of the risk approach is sometimes in danger of obscuring the fact that the chances of the future event (the adverse outcome) actually occurring in a particular person are relatively limited (see Annex 2). However, the predictive power of a risk factor (or combination of risk factors) may well be strong enough to support the various uses suggested in this book. It is very important that the proper use of the risk approach should not spread alarm among those at high relative risk. With these reservations, there seems little doubt that the approach can be used in all the different applications described above and in many other components of primary health care. However, it is important that, whenever possible, the extent of its contribution should be studied and measured operationally. To do this three "facilitating steps" will be required. First, a series of simple research designs must be made available which will provide unequivocal results and from which generalizations can be made.[1] Next, the technical and statistical/epidemiological concepts underlying the risk approach must be made understandable to nonspecialists (the difference between "understanding" and "being able to carry out" is important, for the latter is not always necessary). Finally, the practical aspects of data acquisition, processing, linkage, tabulation and testing must be greatly simplified.

A number of other, more technical, problems must also be solved prior to testing the approach in such vital fields as, for example, the mental health of the family, collaboration with tropical disease control programmes, the planning of social policy, and health worker training. An example would be the validity of the attributable risk, a potentially important tool for social policy of which the limitations are not yet clear. Another example would be the problems associated with calculating the relative risk to whole populations and communities from risk factors such as poverty and illiteracy—another tool of health policy. Other examples would be the desirability, from the ethical point of view, as well as the practicability, of constituting "control" groups for the evaluation of health care in the developing world and the statistical significance of indicators of progress towards health for all. These and many more problems are unlikely to be solved immediately because there is a shortage of the necessary skills. In the search for a way around this apparent impasse, a challenging paradox is encountered. It is to be found as an extension of the fashionable rejection of high technology in health care in the developing world. This rejection is understandable in cases where sophisticated equipment and large hospitals drain scarce resources from the primary level of care, but it is conceivable that the problems of research design and data handling and control in the evaluation of innovations in primary health care are only soluble on the scale needed through technological resourcefulness. Experience with inexpensive, portable, battery-operated microcomputers capable of accommodating all the data handling required—that is, preprogrammed for the complete evaluation project—is therefore urgently required.

Another way of overcoming the familiar shortage of skills needed for the effective monitoring and evaluation of progress in primary health care is to institute an urgent training programme to strengthen the national capability in appropriate health systems research, such as that currently under way in connexion with the risk approach in maternal and child health, including family planning. (A number of workshops on research methods in the evaluation of the risk approach have recently been held in each of the WHO regions.)

---

[1] This approach to health systems research (sometimes described as the "cookbook approach") is of increasing importance as the need to improve health care overtakes the supply of suitably qualified research workers.

8.2 Impediments and Barriers

Some of the problems which have been encountered in the development, implementation and testing of the risk approach in maternal and child health and family planning will have become obvious from the steps described above. They fall into 7 overlapping groups. A few are quite intractable, others are relatively easy to overcome, while yet others have stimulated novel solutions and new insights.

8.2.1 Ethical problems

"No research without service" is more than a slogan; it is an ethical imperative, and the increase in health care coverage during the course of a preliminary population screening for risk is a good example of such a service. What is not so simple, at least from an ethical point of view, is to decide where to stop—in other words, to judge at what point the limited screening for risk is liable to be transformed into a comprehensive screening to determine all the health needs of the individual. Few countries have the necessary resources for this latter procedure, and where it has been tried the results have been disappointing.

Other ethical problems are the impropriety of using a control group in places where there are unmet needs for care, or the deprivation of low-risk mothers and children as a result of reallocating the limited resources available to those at high risk. In some early writing on screening (*30*) a further ethical dilemma was emphasized. A case was made for not screening at all unless full facilities existed for all the treatment that might be required.

8.2.2 Sociological/anthropological problems

The reluctance of some populations to use health care facilities, even when the cost in child mortality is high, is not clearly understood. The impact of Western medicine on indigenous cultures and practices is often counterproductive in this way and the clash of cultures is something to be studied with care (and comprehension) rather than resisted. Working for better health from *within the culture* is not only a principle of the Alma-Ata Declaration, it is probably the only way in which innovations can be successfully introduced. To understand the culture, the skills and insights of the behavioural sciences are needed. In this respect, research workers—particularly medical research workers—have a long way to go, since their formal training does not usually provide such knowledge.

8.2.3 Problems of human motivation

Linked to the difficulties mentioned above are a number of motivational problems which betray "unusual" reasons for apparently irrational behaviour in service or research situations. These reasons are often connected with prestige, status systems, ethnicity, politics, etc., and can complicate and confuse the studies and block innovations. It is unwise to assume the existence of a local reverence for "scientific truth", and different members of the innovating team will probably not share the same motives. An example would be the overriding importance attached to losing face in some cultures where such an effect may, for example, be the result of a low response rate for interviews, the cause of which could have nothing to do with the interviewer.

8.2.4 Political problems

Innovation in health care systems is always difficult—health being such an emotive subject—but it is more than usually difficult where headmen, counsellors or representatives cannot, for political reasons, afford a policy failure or where there is a conflict of ideas within a responsible administration.

The political pressures which play on all members of an innovating team and on responsible officials up to ministry level—and above—are such that a major part of the early planning must be political planning and a major part of the early work must be designed to ensure political support—preferably guaranteed and preferably from above downwards.

8.2.5 Managerial problems

Since the risk approach offers management new tools with which to reorganize and strengthen its own services, representatives of management must at all times be active members of the team, as much involved as possible and always taking part in decision-making. A characteristic problem likely to be encountered is that, in the course of the innovation (and particularly when the local health care system is under scrutiny), major defects in the system will be revealed and, perforce, documented. These discoveries (for example, that the services of trained midwives are rarely solicited, while untrained traditional birth attendants are unfailingly used by local women) seriously threaten those in charge of services. Every effort must be made to protect such persons, and to support them when they draw correct conclusions from the data. Another example of a managerial problem is when a decision has been made to redistribute staff and equipment (to facilitate more rational referral) and this decision is challenged by local representatives of health professional associations. Managers, it will be said, have a difficult enough time as it is, without adding to their problems by introducing changes in patterns of care which, by their nature, cannot be sure of success. Finally, it should be noted that in many countries health care managers are not adequately trained, very poorly paid and without real job tenure. Their feeling of insecurity is therefore justifiable.

8.2.6 Technical problems

Some of these have already been mentioned, but in general it may be said that the design of innovations in health care which derive from the use of risk data is difficult even in highly organized societies with highly organized health care systems. The translation of these models to the developing world (where the need is greatest) presents formidable problems of method. How "scientific" is it possible to be in a poor rural community? How much statistical rigour is attainable? How accurate are the vital data collected in, for example, a region where stillbirth and perinatal death are not notifiable, where the birth of a male is more likely to be registered than that of a female, where the assigning of a cause of death is a matter of lay judgement, or where accidents or maternal deaths, say, are attributed to hostile supernatural forces? It is in just such a society, with its massive burden of illness and its restricted resources, that the need for a risk approach is imperative. Here, therefore, is a major technical problem that involves the simplification of methods and that urgently awaits solution.[1]

8.2.7 Shortage of skilled human resources

The current training programme of WHO recognizes the world shortage of people who can carry out health systems research and seeks to strengthen national and regional capacities in this field. A major difficulty is that of level of skill, since, at the highest level of research design and statistical control, senior epidemiologists and statisticians are needed. Such personnel cannot be trained in a 2-week workshop, though their support staff can. The existing training programmes in the use of the risk approach are therefore of considerable potential value. However, they do not solve the major problem—that is, how to deal with the situation obtaining in areas of the developing world in which the magnitude of need contrasts with the paucity of research skills. Unattractive though the concept is to many health workers, it may still be necessary to standardize methods and produce a packaged set of instructions for the use of the risk approach in health care in which the major statistical and epidemiological exercises are greatly simplified.

8.3 Redressing Inequalities in Health: a Strategy for Improving Primary Health Care

Lessons from early explorations of the risk approach suggest several ways in which it can be applied to improve both the effectiveness and the efficiency of care. An indication has also been given of its resilience, adaptability and capacity to promote concern among those participating. It is an approach with three salient characteristics which commend it particularly as a source of innovation in the implementation of primary health care.

---

[1] One of the most vital problems is to know how general of application are risk factors and scores, and thus to determine how realistic it is to look forward to the day when the risk approach can be reduced to an appropriate and relatively simple form for immediate use with limited need for outside advice.

—*First*, risk is a proxy for need and the risk approach quantifies and guides preventive medicine in a way which can be used by everyone both inside and outside the health care system. It therefore facilitates involvement of the people in health work.

—*Second*, since it aims to provide more care where the need is greatest, it discriminates positively and attacks differentially inequalities in health.

—*Third*, it opens the way to the quantification of the multisectoral contributions to illness represented by poor education, crowding, malnutrition and poverty, and thus, for the first time, makes possible a quantified policy aimed at redressing these major causes of ill health.

If the risk approach can help in these three ways then, with the commitment of governments and people to health, its further use and the measurement of the extent of its contribution become a matter of urgency in the context of primary health care and health for all by the year 2000.

References

1. BUTLER, N. R. & BONHAM, D. G. *Perinatal mortality. The first report of the 1958 British Perinatal Mortality Survey*, Edinburgh and London, Livingstone, 1963.
2. ILLICH, I. *Medical nemesis—the expropriation of health*, London, Calder & Boyars, 1975.
3. MCKEOWN, T. *The role of medicine: dream, mirage or nemesis?* London, Nuffield Provincial Hospitals Trust, 1976.
4. MARTINI, C. J. M. ET AL. *International journal of heatlh services*, **7**: 293 (1977).
5. MAHLER, H. *Scientific American*, **243**: 62 (1980).
6. HUNT, S. M. ET AL. *Journal of epidemiology and community health*, **34**: 281 (1980).
7. WHO Technical Report Series, No. 600, 1976 (*New trends and approaches in the delivery of maternal and child care*: Sixth report of the WHO Expert Committee on Maternal and Child Health).
8. WORLD HEALTH ORGANIZATION. *Alma-Ata 1978. Primary health care. Report of the International Conference on Primary Health Care, Alma-Ata, USSR, 6–12 September 1978 . . .*, Geneva, 1978 ("Health for All" Series, No. 1).
9. DOWIE, J. & LEFRERE, P., ed. *Risk and chance*, Milton Keynes, The Open University Press, 1980.
10. HAYNES, R. B. ET AL. *New England journal of medicine*, **299**: 741 (1978).
11. AYER, A. J. In: DOWIE, J. & LEFRERE, P., ed. *Risk and chance*, Milton Keynes, The Open University Press, 1980.
12. DOLL, R. & PETO, R. *Journal of the National Cancer Institute*, **66**: 1191 (1981).
13. BUTLER, N. R. & ALBERMAN, E. The effects of smoking in pregnancy. In: *Perinatal problems. The second report of the 1958 British Perinatal Mortality Survey*, Edinburgh and London, Livingstone, 1969.
14. SUSSER, M. *Causal thinking in the health sciences: concepts and strategies of epidemiology*, London, Oxford University Press, 1980.
15. LILIENFELD, A. M. & LILIENFELD, D. E. *Foundations of epidemiology*, 2nd ed., New York, Oxford University Press, 1980.
16. BARKER, D. J. P. & ROSE, G. *Epidemiology in medical practice*, Edinburgh, Churchill Livingstone, 2nd ed., 1979, p. 76.
17. MCMAHON, B. & PUGH, T. F. *Epidemiology; principles and methods*, Boston, Little, Brown, 1970.
18. WALTER, S. D. *Biometrics*, **32**: 829 (1976).
19. LEVIN, M. L. *Acta; Unio internationalis contra cancrum*, **19**: 531 (1953).
20. SCOTT, A. ET AL. *European journal of obstetrics, gynaecology and reproductive biology*, **12**: 157 (1981).
21. Relative or attributable risk. *Lancet*, **2**: 1211 (1981).
22. ARMITAGE, P. *Statistical methods in medical research*, Oxford, Blackwell Scientific Publications, 1971.
23. HODGETTS, R. M. *Management: theory, process and practice*, Philadelphia, London, and Toronto, Saunders, 1975.
24. MOONEY, G. ET AL. *Choices for health care*, London, Macmillan, 1980, app. 5.

25. WORLD HEALTH ORGANIZATION. *Global Strategy for health for all by the year 2000*, Geneva, 1981, pp. 62, 63 ("Health for All" Series, No. 3).
26. ROSE, G. *Tidsskift for den Norske Laegerforening*, **101**: 722 (1981).
27. WORLD HEALTH ORGANIZATION. *The managerial process for national health development. Guiding principles for use in support of strategies for health for all by the year 2000*, Geneva, 1981 ("Health for All" Series, No. 5).
28. NEWELL, K. W., ed. *Health by the people*, Geneva, World Health Organization, 1975.
29. WORLD HEALTH ORGANIZATION. *Development of indicators for monitoring progress towards health for all by the year 2000*, Geneva, 1981 ("Health for All" Series, No. 4).
30. WILSON, J. M. G. & JUNGNER, G. *The principles and practice of screening for disease*, Geneva, World Health Organization, 1968 (Public Health Papers, No. 34).

Acknowledgements

The WHO Risk Approach Task Force (of which the authors were Chairman, Rapporteur, and Secretary, respectively) was responsible for the development of the early applications of the strategy to maternal and child health care and family planning and contributed to the preparation of *Risk approach for maternal and child health care* (WHO Offset Publication No. 39, Geneva, World Health Organization, 1978)—the predecessor of the present book. The authors are indebted to the following persons, who constituted the other members of the Task Force:

Dr N. Butler, Royal Hospital for Sick Children, Bristol, England
Dr N. H. Fisek, Director, Institute of Community Medicine, Hacettepe University, Ankara, Turkey
Dr H. Goldstein, Professor of Statistics, University of London Institute of Education, London, England
Dr R. Karim, Deputy Director of Health Services (MCH), Ministry of Health, Kuala Lumpur, Malaysia
Dr Z. K. Stembera, Research Institute for the Care of Mother and Child, Prague, Czechoslovakia.

Thanks are also due to Dr E. Liisberg, Dr B. McCarthy, and Ms E. Royston, of the Division of Family Health, WHO, for their helpful comments and suggestions, as well as to Ms D. Erstling, of the same division, who, in addition to assisting in the preparation of this book, contributed the list of annotated references in Annex 3 which were selected from a bibliography that she herself compiled.

The World Health Organization gratefully acknowledges the financial support of the United Nations Fund for Population Activities.

Annexes

Annex 1

Selecting target health problems

Among the many health problems afflicting mothers and children, it is usually a simple matter to choose the "most important". However, this choice is often coloured by the opinions of those who make it and may not be correct from the point of view of the local community. Nor does it always reflect the essential facts about health or their trends in time. Finally, the "most important" health problems are not always the best targets for prevention, because in some instances they present greater difficulties and require the expenditure of many more resources than do other health problems. To weigh these considerations in the balance and to facilitate the process of establishing an order of priority for health problems a number of techniques have been evolved. The notes below summarize one of the simplest methods. Using a simple rating scale, it balances the sometimes conflicting factors of prevalence, seriousness, preventability, trends in time, and local concern.

The method, which uses weighted criteria, starts from the assumption that, in different places, a rough estimate can be made (on, say, a 4- or

Example:

Health problem	Criterion	Maximum possible rating	Rate accorded
Maternal mortality	Extent	10	3
	Seriousness	10	10
	Preventability	10	8
	Local concern	10	10
	Time trend	10	2
Neonatal tetanus	Extent	10	8
	Seriousness	10	10
	Preventability	10	10
	Local concern	10	4
	Time trend	10	5
Childhood road accidents	Extent	10	3
	Seriousness	10	10
	Preventability	10	5
	Local concern	10	7
	Time trend	10	8

5-point scale) as to the relative importance, or weight, to be accorded to the different aspects of a health problem—namely, its prevalence, its seriousness, its preventability, its trend in time, and how it is regarded locally. In addition, it is assumed that each health problem, such as maternal mortality, neonatal tetanus or childhood road accidents, can be rated (this time perhaps on a 10-point scale) on each of the above aspects, or criteria. (See example on preceding page.)

The relative importance of each criterion will already have been given a weight—say, on a 5-point scale—so that perhaps the extent and seriousness of a problem are both considered vital and given 5, while preventability is given less—say, 3—along with local concern. Time trend is deemed to matter least and is given a weight of 2.

A simple matrix will set the health problems in an order of priority, as follows:

Health problem	Extent (weight 5)	Serious- ness (weight 5)	Prevent- ability (weight 3)	Local concern (weight 3)	Time trend (weight 2)	Total score
1. Maternal mortality	(3 ×5)	(10 ×5)	(8 ×3)	(10 ×3)	(2 ×2)	123
2. Neonatal tetanus	(8 ×5)	(10 ×5)	(10 ×3)	(4 ×3)	(5 ×2)	142
3. Childhood road accidents	(3 ×5)	(10 ×5)	(5 ×3)	(7 ×3)	(8 ×2)	117

Criteria and relative weights

The order of priority would therefore be: first, neonatal tetanus; second, maternal mortality; and third, childhood road accidents. A scrutiny of the matrix might well lead to the use of different ratings, and so in theory any priority could be accorded to any problem. The value of the method therefore lies in its ability to force consideration of the major factors in decision-making and in its use of data, no matter how crude, whenever possible.

Annex 2

A note on risk measurements

Relative Risk

As has been indicated in Chapter 3 of the main text (section 3.3.2, p. 21), the relative risk is the incidence of a particular disease or cause of death in a population exposed to or with the relevant risk factor divided by the corresponding morbidity or mortality in a population not exposed to or without the risk factor. For this reason it is sometimes called the "risk ratio". Care must be taken in calculating morbidity and mortality rates from various kinds of data, and the methods—as well as the pitfalls—are dealt with in Chapter 8 of *Foundations of epidemiology*, by Lilienfeld & Lilienfeld.[1]

Attributable Risk

This measure of association is also well described in Chapter 8 of *Foundations of epidemiology*. Some confusion may arise through the use of different terminology (for example, "risk difference," "rate difference", "etiologic fraction") by other authors.

Lilienfeld & Lilienfeld define attributable risk (following Levin on lung cancer[2]) as the maximum proportion of the total morbidity or mortality in the population attributable to the risk factor. It brings together the relative risk and the proportion of the population with the risk factor. The formula used (the derivation of which is also described in *Foundations of epidemiology*) is:

$$\frac{b(y-1)}{b(y-1)+1}$$

where b is the proportion of the population with the risk factor and y is the relative risk associated with that factor.

The standard error and confidence limits of this expression must be

---

[1] Lilienfeld, A. M. & Lilienfeld, D. E. *Foundations of epidemiology*, 2nd ed., New York, Oxford University Press, 1980.
[2] Levin, M. L. *Acta, Unio internationalis contra cancrum*, **19**: 531 (1953).

respected as must the underlying assumptions, of which the most important is that of causality. There is also the assumption (though only in the background in some of the literature) that, apart from the risk factor under scrutiny, other causally related risk factors are equally distributed in the whole population. The attributable risk can be computed for multiple as well as single factors.

Example 1

Annex Table 1 presents a classic table derived from the British Perinatal Survey of 1958, to which figures for relative and attributable risks have been added. Their value, as additions to the conventional presentation of data, may be judged by reference to Table 2, in Chapter 2 of the main text (page 16).

Example 2

Annex Table 2 illustrates an example taken from the paper by Scott et al.,[1] who explored the relative and attributable risks associated with 8 maternal risk factors for small-for-gestational-age (SGA) babies—a proxy for many major perinatal problems.

The most important risk factor among multiparous women was the slow intrauterine growth rate of previous offspring. Previous slow growth was associated with a relative risk of nearly 8 and an attributable risk of 56% for an SGA baby. The attributable risk of all 8 factors together was about 88%.

One important finding of this study was that adjustment for maternal height and weight, smoking habits, "pathological factors" and sibling birth weight satisfactorily accounted for the well-known "social class" effect in the distribution of SGA babies.

Predictive Power (or Value)

The positive predictive power, or predictive power of a positive test for the risk factor, is the probability that a person with that risk factor later turns out to experience the unwanted outcome. The negative predictive power, or predictive power of a negative test (or the absence of the risk factor), is the probability that a person without that risk factor turns out not to experience the unwanted outcome. So the positive predictive power of the test for the risk factor shown in Table 3, in Chapter 3 of the main text (p. 30), is as follows:

$$\frac{\text{True positives}}{\text{All those with the risk factor (i.e., true positives + false positives)}} = \frac{200}{200 + 50} = 80\%$$

---

[1] Scott, A. et al. *European journal of obstetrics, gynaecology and reproductive biology*, **12**: 157 (1981).

ANNEX 2

Annex Table 1. Perinatal death rates (per 1000 live births) by cause in 7 high-risk groups: all births, England, Scotland, and Wales, March 1958*

| Risk factors | Percentage of all births | Cause of death ||||||| Relative risk | Attributable risk (%) |
		Congenital abnormality	Antepartum deaths	Perinatal hypoxia	Birth trauma	Immaturity	Infections	Other causes	All causes		
1. Mother, parity 4+	8.9	7.4	9.6	12.6	5.5	4.1	2.4	10.2	51.8	1.65	4
2. Mother single	2.9	7.8	8.8	8.8	3.8	4.9	3.4	6.4	43.9	1.34	1
3. Father unskilled	9.3	8.4	6.8	9.9	3.3	4.1	2.1	7.6	42.2	1.31	3
4. Severe pre-eclampsia in pregnancy	5.6	6.1	26.5	18.2	6.3	7.8	2.5	12.6	80.0	2.63	8
5. Spontaneous breech	2.2	42.4	48.9	46.3	29.3	23.4	3.9	39.8	244.5	8.60	6
6. Vaginal bleeding before 28th week of gestation	2.9	7.2	10.6	12.1	4.8	24.2	3.9	12.5	75.3	2.36	4
7. Antepartum haemorrhage	0.4	21.4	67.9	314.3	21.4	57.1	14.3	35.7	557.1	17.92	6
All births 3–9 March 1958 (Total = 16 994)	100.0	5.8	6.8	7.1	3.1	3.3	1.5	5.6	33.2	1.0	

* Source: Butler, N. R. & Bonham, D. G. *Perinatal mortality. The first report of the 1958 British Perinatal Mortality Survey*, Edinburgh and London, Livingstone, 1963.

Annex Table 2. The relative and attributable risks associated with 8 risk factors identified in the reproductive performance of mothers of 488 small-for-gestational-age babies and 367 average-for-gestational-age babies in Oxford, England, 1964–77*

Risk factors	Relative risk[a]	Attributable risk
1. Weight of previous liveborn siblings (below −1 S.D.)	7.98 (4.7–13.5)	56.0% (46.9–63.5)
2. Smoking	3.04 (2.2–4.2)	39.7% (32.9–45.8)
3. Hypertension without pre-eclampsia	2.84 (1.9–4.2)	18.4% (12.5–24.0)
4. Pre-eclampsia	15.78 (6.2–40.4)	9.8% (6.4–13.1)
5. Maternal height (below −1 S.D.)	2.03 (1.3–3.1)	15.8% (9.0–22.0)
6. Maternal weight (below −1 S.D.)	1.84 (1.2–2.8)	13.8% (6.6–20.5)
7. Net pregnancy weight gain (below −1 S.D.)	1.78 (1.1–2.8)	10.2% (3.3–16.6)
8. Manual social class	1.08 (0.8–1.5)	5.2% (−15.8–22.4)

* Source: Scott et al., *op. cit.*

Notes: [a] Numbers in parentheses are confidence limits.
All births were singletons and congenital abnormality was excluded.
Confounding or overlap between risk factors was taken into consideration.

In Table 3 the occurrence of the unwanted outcome in the population of mothers is 225/1000, or 1 in 4.4 (this is the number of unwanted outcomes that one would expect if the total population of mothers were 1000) and the chances of a positive test are 250/1000, or 1 in 4. The chances of the test results being incorrect are 1 in 5, and, conversely, the chances of their being correct are 4 in 5. But the population subjected to the test may not be representative of the total population of mothers, among whom the outcome might be much less frequent.

Care must therefore be taken to ensure that, in calculating probabilities, the incidence of the outcome in the population is taken into consideration as well as the quality of the test for the risk factor. The relationship between these elements—and a way of calculating the predictive power of the test for the whole population (if screening test results for the total are not available)—is given by:

$$\text{Positive predictive power} = \frac{(Se)(P)}{(Se)(P) + (1 - Sp)(1 - P)}$$

where Se = how good the test is at selecting those who will suffer the unwanted outcome—that is:

$$\frac{\text{true positives}}{\text{total who suffer the unwanted outcome}}$$

Sp = how good the test is at selecting those who will avoid the unwanted outcome—that is:

$$\frac{\text{true negatives}}{\text{total who avoid the unwanted outcome}}$$

$P =$ the prevalence (or, where that is not available or not relevant, the incidence) of the unwanted outcome in the total population.

Further Examples of Risk Factors which Can Be Ascertained without the Use of Advanced Technology

Perinatal mortality

In Barron's series from Indonesia[1] the main risk factors appeared to be as follows:

(1) *Low birth weight* (36% of the perinatal deaths)

Main risk factors:

—Mother aged under 17 years or 35 years or more

—Low prepregnancy weight

—Poor maternal weight gain

—Grand multiparity

—Short interpregnancy interval

—Previous pregnancy loss

—Multiple pregnancy

—Vaginal bleeding

—"Pre-eclampsia"

—Previous induced abortion

—Chronic infection

—Smoking

—Short stature

Tools and procedures needed for screening:

Questionnaire, paper, pencil, weighing apparatus, instrument for blood-pressure measurement, tape measure.

---

[1] Barron, S. L. *Journal of obstetrics and gynaecology of the British Commonwealth*, **81**: 187 (1974).

(2) *Birth trauma* (18% of the perinatal deaths)

Main risk factors:

—Cephalopelvic disproportion

—Previous babies over 4 kg in weight

—Previous deliveries necessitating surgical intervention

—Previous unattended labour

Tools and procedures needed for screening:

Questionnaire, paper, pencil; clinical examination for cephalopelvic disproportion.

(3) *Fetal hypoxia* (13% of the perinatal deaths)

Main risk factors:

—Mother over 35 years of age

—Maternal malnutrition

—Grand multiparity

—Maternal obesity

—Previous perinatal death

—Anaemia

—Chronic infections—e.g., malaria

—Poor weight gain

—Vaginal bleeding

—"Pre-eclampsia"

—Chronic diseases: diabetes, cardiorenal, etc.

—Multiple pregnancy

—Breech presentation

—Placenta previa

Tools and procedures needed for screening:

Questionnaire, paper, pencil, weighing apparatus, instrument for blood-pressure measurement, urine and blood testing apparatus; clinical examination.

(4) *Antepartum haemorrhage* (10% of perinatal deaths)

Main risk factors:

—History of trauma

— "Pre-eclampsia"
— Other hypertension
— Multiple pregnancy

Tools and procedures needed for screening:

Questionnaire, paper, pencil, instrument for blood-pressure measurement; clinical examination.

Infant and toddler mortality[1]

(1) *Protein-energy deficiency* (12% of deaths)

Main risk factors:

— Parental illiteracy
— Mother working away from home
— Lack of breast-feeding
— Poor feeding patterns
— Short interpregnancy interval
— History of diarrhoea
— History of measles
— History of pertussis

(2) *Pneumonia* (12% of deaths)

Main risk factors:
— History of upper respiratory disease
— History of diarrhoea

(3) *Diarrhoea* (12% of deaths)

Main risk factors:
— Artificial feeding
— Malnutrition
— Polluted drinking-water
— Flies
— Inadequate disposal of faeces

---

[1] Morley, D. *Paediatric priorities in the developing world*, London, Butterworth, 1973 (Postgraduate Paediatric Series).

—Poor personal hygiene

—History of measles

(4) *Measles* (8% of deaths)

Main risk factors:

—Malnutrition

—Overcrowding

(5) *Pertussis* (8% of deaths)

Main risk factors:

—Malnutrition

—Overcrowding

Tools and procedures needed for screening causes (1)–(5):

Questionnaire, paper, pencil.

NOTE: Most of the above risk factors will be universal and though their relative and attributable risks will vary from place to place it is probably reasonable, where surveys cannot be done locally, to take over major groupings of risk factors and related scores from risk research projects in comparable areas. Interventions after screening and scoring will be along the lines described in Chapter 5 and will follow the priorities dictated by the relative and attributable risks associated with the risk factors.

A Further Note on Scoring

It has been recommended that if the scoring of risk is to be used in individual care, the relative risk should be the basis of the score. If communities and their services are the object of attention, then both the distribution of the relative risks in that community and the attributable risks would be the starting-points for change.

These scoring methods have not invariably been used; Annex Tables 3, 4 and 5 show examples of rather more complex methods. In the first two the risk score is adjusted to represent what would happen without intervention—that is, the probable incidence of the unwanted outcome. In the third, the occurrence of the risk factor in mothers experiencing the unwanted outcome is the measure used.

To convert the scores for use, they were added and then, by reference to a conversion table, produced as if they were perinatal death rates. Thus a score of −500 would be expected to indicate a perinatal death rate of 15.4 per 1000, a score of zero a rate of 34.9 per 1000 and a score of +500 a rate of 65.5 per 1000.

Annex Table 3. A scoring system based on data from the 1958 British Perinatal Survey (16 994 births)*

Risk factors	Subgroups of risk factors used	Risk score
Maternal age	Under 35 years	−138
	35 years and over	+138
Parity	0	+29
	1–3	−98
	4+	+69
Social class[a]	I and II	−84
	III	+8
	IV and V	+76
Maternal height	Under 157 cm	+62
	157 cm or more	−62
Pre-eclampsia	None to moderate	−280
	Severe	+280
Cigarette-smoking	Smokers	+85
	Nonsmokers	−85

* Source: Butler, N. R. & Alberman, E. D. *Perinatal problems. The second report of the 1958 British Perinatal Survey*, chapter 3, Edinburgh and London, Livingstone, 1969. (See also Appendix Table 1.)

[a] A socioeconomic classification based on partner's occupation.

In Annex Table 4, the scores presented are the result of a complex standardization procedure, which, like the scoring shown in Annex Table 3, indicates a perinatal death rate that would probably be experienced if no further action were taken.

Reconciling Scores, Care and Resources

The "trade-off" of need for care against the resources available has been mentioned in Chapter 4 of the main text (sections 4.1.2 and 4.1.3, pp. 36–38). To obtain the best possible reconciliation of scores (representing need for care) and available resources, economists use the notions of the marginal costs and benefits involved at each score level. In theory, the optimum balance will be struck when the ratios of the expected marginal benefits to marginal costs are equalized: that is, when

$$\frac{MBa}{MCa} = \frac{MBb}{MCb} \quad \frac{MBc}{MCc} = \text{a constant}$$

where MB = marginal benefits
MC = marginal costs
for: a = high scores; b = medium scores; c = low scores.

Thus, MCa is the marginal cost of the care needed by high scores, MCb the cost of that needed by medium scores, and MCc the cost of that needed by low scores.

The corresponding marginal benefits (MBa, MBb and MBc) are measured by assigning monetary values to the results of the care (the expected decline in perinatal or maternal mortality, for example). If the resources available are fixed, then the levels of care assigned to the scores will have to be adjusted until the ratios become constant.[1]

Annex Table 4. A scoring system based on data from the Jerusalem Perinatal Survey (42 002 singleton births between 1966 and 1972); risk score for the total population = 15*

Risk factors	Subgroups of risk factors used	Risk score[a]
Maternal age	Under 40 years	–
	40 years and over	22
Maternal age and parity	Primiparae aged 35 or more	22
	Others	–
Multiple pregnancy and parity	Twin pregnancy primiparae	133
	Twin pregnancy multiparae	40
Previous pregnancy loss	Previous stillbirth	91
Previous child loss	Previous child death	24
Pre-eclampsia	Present or not known	77
	Absent	–
Diabetes	"Pre-diabetes"	28
	Diabetes	77

* Source: Davies, A. M. & Harlap, S. *Antenatal prediction of peri- and neonatal mortality risk*. (Paper presented at the Consultation on Identification and Assessment of High Risk for Development of Intervention Strategies in Maternal and Child Care, including Family Planning, 10–16 December 1974, Geneva, World Health Organization; unpublished document MCH/WP/HR/74.1).

[a] The risk score in this case is the predicted perinatal death rate.

---

[1] See the section on marginal analysis in: Mooney, G. et al. *Choices for health care*, London, Macmillan, 1980.

Annex Table 5. The scoring of risk by frequency of risk factor in women delivering low-birth-weight babies: a comparison of the outcomes "prematurity" and "small for date"*

Risk factors	Frequency of risk factor, compared with normal controls, in mothers whose babies were:	
	"Premature"	"Small for date"
Age under 18 years	2.8	–
Previous induced abortion	1.8	–
Unmarried	1.8	–
Moderate to severe toxaemia of pregnancy	1.7	3.0
History of renal disease	1.7	2.4
History of perinatal loss	1.7	–
Previous sterility	1.5	2.4
First-trimester bleeding	1.4	2.0
Age over 30 years	1.3	1.2
Height less than 155 cm	–	4.3
Mild toxaemia of pregnancy	–	1.4
Pregnancy weight increase less than 7 kg	–	1.4

* Source: Stembera, Z. K. *Factors influencing length of gestation and fetal growth (etiology of low birth weight)*, Geneva, World Health Organization, 1975 (unpublished document MCH/LBW/WP 75.3).

Note: This paper was particularly concerned with the mother–child interaction.

Annex 3

Annotated bibliography*

AKHTAR, J. & SEGHAL, N. Prognostic value of a prepartum and intrapartum risk-scoring method. *Southern medical journal*, **73**: 411–414 (1980).

A simple prepartum and intrapartum scoring technique for the identification of high-risk patients was evaluated. A modification of the risk-scoring form of Coopland et al. was applied to 1224 obstetric patients at the Charleston Area Medical Center, Charleston, SC, USA. Patients were scored on three occasions: at the time of the initial visit, on admission to the labour suite, and at delivery. They were classified as being at low, moderate or high risk, according to the total risk score. Of the 147 patients (12.1%) who were considered at high risk at the time of delivery, 114 (77.62%) were so designated at the initial scoring, indicating that most high-risk patients can be identified at their first evaluation. Risk status, as determined by this scoring method, was related to the following outcome measures: type of delivery, selected intrapartum complications, perinatal mortality, 5-minute Apgar scores and nursery care of the newborn, and length of gestation.

Of all perinatal deaths, 70% occurred in the 25% of patients identified as moderate and high risk, indicating that this scoring method effectively identified high-risk prenatal patients.

ALBERMAN, E. & GOLDSTEIN, H. The "at-risk" register: a statistical evaluation. *British journal of preventive and social medicine*, **24**: 129–135 (1970).

A system of selective screening of children at high risk of handicapping conditions not apparent at birth was assessed. On the basis of an analysis of data from the National Child Development Study, United Kingdom, on 12 083 births, it was found that the statistically significant predictors of handicap were parity, method of delivery and neonatal illness.

A mathematical model was proposed to determine the allocation of resources among children at different risk of handicap, so that the maximum number of handicaps would be detected. The authors suggested dividing births into high- and low-risk groups, and to differentiate between these groups in allocating resources for detecting handicaps. Only in areas where the detection rate is

---

* Selected from an annotated bibliography entitled "Risk Approach for Maternal and Child Health" (document MCH/RA/81–1), which is available, on request, from: Maternal and Child Health, Division of Family Health, World Health Organization, 1211 Geneva 27, Switzerland.

exceedingly low is it advisable to concentrate all resources on the high-risk group. In all other areas, it is preferable to devote a proportion of the resources to the remaining children, a proportion which should increase as the basic detection rate rises. The authors emphasized that to achieve the best possible use of resources, continuous review of the existing situation is necessary.

BARRON, S. L. Perinatal mortality and birthweight in Makassar, Indonesia. *Journal of obstetrics and gynaecology of the British Commonwealth*, **81**: 187–195 (1974).

On the basis of data collected in 1969 at 2 hospitals in Makassar, Indonesia, cause of perinatal mortality was examined for 1333 perinatal deaths out of 48 582 live births from 1951 to 1969. Causes of death were compared with those in the 1958 British Perinatal Mortality Survey (first report). A separate study of birth weight was carried out on 1060 infants born in 1969. Results (adjusted for differences in social class, maternal stature and birth order) showed that Chinese Indonesian infants had a higher mean birth weight than did non-Chinese Indonesian infants.

BUTLER, W. R. & ALBERMAN E. D. High-risk predictors at booking and in pregnancy. In: *Perinatal problems*, Edinburgh, Livingstone, 1969, pp. 36–46.

The effect of combined factors (smoking, pre-eclamptic toxaemia, antepartum haemorrhage and low haemoglobin) on pregnancy in women of different characteristics (age, parity, height, socioeconomic status, region and place of delivery) was determined using data from the United Kingdom on singleton births during 1 week and stillbirths and neonatal deaths during a 3-month period.

Detailed explanations of the statistical methods used to study the various combinations of maternal characteristics at booking, together with a description of conditions occurring subsequently, are provided. A statistical appendix (by H. Goldstein) includes discussion of several possible mathematical models.

DISSEVELT, A. G. ET AL. An antenatal record card for identification of high risk cases by auxiliary midwives at rural health centres. *Tropical and geographical medicine*, **28**: 251–255 (1976).

The use of a prenatal record card to facilitate the selection of high-risk cases by midwives in rural health centres in Kenya was described. The record card, in effect since 1972, was designed for use with manuals of standards of care. The selection of criteria for predicting risk, as well as the determination of cut-off points for each criterion, was discussed.

Special features of the card included: built-in warning system to identify high-risk cases, indications for decision-making on type of care to be given, use during several pregnancies, and compactness.

Midwives who worked with the card stated that it facilitated their work. Improvement in the quality of prenatal care was attributed to use of the record card in an assessment carried out under the auspices of the Kenya–Netherlands Project for Operations Research in Outpatient Services.

EDWARDS, L. E. ET AL. A simplified antepartum risk-scoring system. *Obstetrics and gynecology*, **54**: 237–240 (1979).

The effectiveness of a simple antepartum risk-scoring system was evaluated in

2085 consecutive deliveries at St Paul Ramsey Hospital and Medical Center, St Paul, MN, USA, during the period 1974–1977. In all, 67 demographic, obstetric, medical and miscellaneous factors were selected for the risk-scoring system. A numerical value was assigned to each factor by considering its potential impact on neonatal morbidity and mortality. Risk scores, obtained for each patient at the first prenatal visit, were updated at 36 weeks' gestation, and, finally, on admission to the hospital for labour and delivery. The final risk score, fetal and neonatal mortality, and neonatal morbidity (defined as any condition requiring admission to the newborn intensive care unit) were recorded; the data were analysed to determine the sensitivity and specificity of the scoring system.

Neonatal morbidity was observed in 42.1% of infants of mothers classified as high risk compared with 12.5% of infants of mothers classified as low risk. No neonatal deaths were observed in the low-risk group; there were 34 in the high-risk group. The perinatal mortality rates for low- and high-risk pregnancies were, respectively, 7.2 and 63.3 per 1000 live births; 88.6% of all perinatal deaths occurred in the high-risk group.

EISNER, V. ET AL. The risk of low birth weight. *American journal of public health*, **69**: 887–893 (1979).

Birth records of 505 243 single live births in the USA during 1974 were analysed to identify the factors associated with a high incidence of low-birth-weight babies. Multivariate analysis was used to determine the correlates of low birth weight. When other factors were held constant, the following factors each increased the risk of having a low-birth-weight infant: race not white, previous reproductive loss, short interpregnancy interval, out-of-wedlock birth, no prenatal care, and maternal age under 18 years or over 35 years. Odds ratios were presented, and the method for combining these to estimate an individual mother's risk of having a low-birth-weight infant was illustrated.

ESSEX, B. & EVERETT, V. Use of an action-oriented record card for antenatal screening. *Tropical doctor*, **7**: 134–138 (1977).

The design and testing of an prenatal record card developed in Dar es Salaam, United Republic of Tanzania, were described. The card was intended to be independent of recall, detect women at risk of complications during labour, indicate the appropriate action for each abnormality detected, emphasize the treatment needed to prevent anaemia, malaria, neonatal tetanus and malnutrition, and provide the mother with a permanent record of risk and the outcome of the pregnancy. Appropriate parameters for identifying women at risk in the study area were established.

To measure the rate at which cases at risk were detected with the use of the prenatal card, a total of 13 410 women who attended 41 mobile prenatal clinics were screened. It was found that the prenatal card had a much higher detection rate than a card that had previously been used. The authors suggested that, with the exception of height and possibly parity, the criteria used in this prenatal card were of universal application in most developing countries. Of the total risk factors, 81% were present throughout pregnancy and would be detected even if the woman was seen only once. The standardization of referral patterns could lead to improved prenatal care.

GRANTHAM-MCGREGOR, S. ET AL. The identification of infants at risk of malnutrition in Kingston, Jamaica. *Tropical and geographical medicine*, **29**: 165–171 (1977).

A longitudinal study was carried out on the growth, health and environment of 270 infants from birth to 1 year of age in Kingston, Jamaica. To determine the factors related to increased risk of malnutrition, the records of children in the 10th percentile for weight at 12 months of age were reviewed to see whether these children differed from the remaining children in their health care or social background.

Of the 8 factors considered, high birth order (over 6), substandard housing, incompetent mothers, repeated attacks of gastroenteritis, poor clinic attendance, poor milk intake and low birth weight were all significantly related to being underweight at 1 year. These factors were interrelated, and the more factors that were present the smaller the child tended to be. The authors stressed the importance of home visiting, both in order to locate children not regularly attending clinics and to assess housing standards and the competence of the mother.

LARSEN, J. & MULLER, E. Obstetric care in a rural population. *South African medical journal*, **54**: 1137–1140 (1978).

A retrospective analysis of 678 randomly selected patients who delivered at Charles Johnson Memorial Hospital, Ngutu, KwaZulu, South Africa, in 1977 was undertaken. Its purpose was to determine both the number of high-risk patients in this rural population and the value of prenatal screening to preselect women requiring hospital delivery, as well as to interpret these findings in terms of the design and function of rural obstetric services.

Over 50% of this population were found to have significant risk factors warranting hospital delivery. The nature of these risk factors was described. Results indicated that 85% of such patients could be detected ante partum; they should be admitted to "waiting mothers areas" before the onset of labour to avoid transport problems and consequent perinatal and maternal mortality. The need for adequate postnatal facilities was also discussed.

MADELEY, R. Relating child health services to needs by the use of simple epidemiology. *Public health*, **92**: 224–230 (1978).

To use health services in the most efficient and effective manner, a method was developed to identify children and families in need of extra help during the first few months of life. Data on 72 children, aged 1 month to 1 year, who died in the Nottingham area, United Kingdom, from 1974 to 1976 were obtained from birth and death notifications, health visitors' records, obstetric records of the mother and an "at-risk" register. Two controls were chosen for each death and similar information was obtained. Chi-square tests were carried out to determine the degree of importance of a particular item as a risk factor. Those items showing a difference significant at the 10% level or higher were investigated further using the method of stepwise discriminant analysis.

MADELEY, R. & LATHAM, A. Management aspects of high risk strategies in child health. *Community medicine*, **1**: 36–39 (1979).

The implementation of a plan in Nottingham, United Kingdom, to concentrate health visitors in areas with high post-neonatal death rates was described. Using a stepwise discriminant analysis based on the death or survival of babies in the post-neonatal period, a risk scoring system was devised including the following factors: born in deprived area or not, birth weight, breast-fed baby or not, maternal age, and duration of second stage of labour. On the basis of their score, babies were assigned to a high-risk category and followed up more intensively. Of 2882 births in Nottingham in the first 5 months of 1978, 344 (12% of total births) were in the high-risk group.

Why certain babies were included for special follow-up while others were not was difficult for some health visitors to understand. Procedures for handling this difficulty were reviewed. Another potential problem—maternal anxiety caused by more frequent health visiting—did not arise.

A method of reallocation was proposed: maintaining services at their present level in the more affluent areas and recruiting new staff for assignment to areas where the needs have been shown to be greatest.

It was found that post-neonatal deaths were grouped in certain parts of the city, and that there was a striking relationship between social deprivation and post-neonatal mortality. The scoring system developed assigned points according to: birth in a deprived area, birth weight, breast-fed baby, maternal age, and second stage of labour less than 15 minutes. With the use of this system, 10% of total births were identified as being at risk, which would correctly identify 55% of deaths. Sensitivity was 53%; specificity was 91%.

NEUTRA, R. A case-control study for estimating the risk of eclampsia in Cali, Colombia. *American journal of obstetrics and gynecology*, **117**: 894–903 (1973).

Two hundred and twenty eclamptic patients were compared with a random sample of 345 patients from the general population of Cali, Colombia, in order to quantify the predictive value of 6 variables which can be determined at the onset of pregnancy: age, parity, number of previous abortions and stillbirths, marital status, social class, and migration status.

Results showed that eclampsia was strongly related to parity and age. Unmarried status and history of previous abortion were also related to eclampsia. The author noted that a risk score based on these 4 variables could predict the 12% of the population which would produce 56% of the eclamptic cases. Age-parity-specific eclampsia rates and crude rates were calculated. These results were compared with data from other countries and differences were discussed.

OSOFSKY, H. J. & KENDALL, N. Poverty as a criterion of risk. *Clinical obstetrics and gynecology*, **16**: 103–119 (1973).

The effects of poverty on pregnancy outcome and child development were reviewed. As an example of the increased risks of the poor, the authors noted that of 1371 patients receiving prenatal care at Temple University Hospital, a facility serving a low-income area in Philadelphia, PA, USA, 47.2% were found to be at high risk as determined by the departmental high-risk classification system. Data concerning pregnancy outcome, including its relation to maternal age, maternal care, and maternal risk status were described.

PERKIN, G. W. Assessment of reproductive risk in nonpregnant women. *American journal of obstetrics and gynecology*, **101**: 709–717 (1968).

A method of assessing reproductive risk in nonpregnant women was devised based on age, parity, medical and obstetric history, birth interval, and socio-economic status. Evidence supporting the relationship of these factors to maternal and infant mortality and morbidity was reviewed.

The scoring system was intended for hospital use to identify the group of postpartum women most likely to be at risk in a subsequent pregnancy. These women would receive contraceptive counselling; the high-risk group would receive intensified follow-up care to ensure that contraception was continued. Use of the scoring system in developing countries was discussed.

PUFFER, R. & SERRANO, C. V. Results of the Inter-American Investigations of Mortality Relating to Reproduction. *Bulletin of the Pan American Health Organization*, **10**: 131–142 (1976).

On the basis of a survey of infant mortality in Latin America, maternal age and parity were shown to have a direct influence on infant health and survival. Immaturity, or low birth weight, and malnutrition were the major underlying causes of death. The importance of considering maternal age, birth order, and birth weight when planning preventive health programmes was stressed. Difficulties in collecting infant mortality data were reviewed and the need for good-quality data was emphasized.

RUMEAU-ROUQUETTE, C. ET AL. Risk indicators and environment-investigations in France. In: *Proceedings of the 8th World Congress of Gynecology and Obstetrics, Mexico City, 1976*. Amsterdam, Excerpta Medica, 1977, pp. 1728–1733.

Risk factors in neonatal pathology were studied in two investigations in France. A prospective study was carried out from 1963 to 1968 in the Paris area on 12 000 pregnant women. In 1972 a nationwide retrospective study of 11 200 representative births was conducted paying special attention to drug use, alcohol consumption, and sociocultural factors.

Statistical analyses indicated that the nature of the risk factor varied with the specific pregnancy outcome. Results were discussed in terms of risks related to the following: stillbirth, prematurity, fetal hypotrophy, acute fetal distress, and congenital malformations. Risk factors were categorized as avoidable, sociocultural and those related to women's attitude towards reproduction. Preventive measures were suggested to reduce these risks.

SHAPIRO, S. ET AL. Relationships of selected prenatal factors to pregnancy outcome and congenital anomalies. *American journal of public health*, **55**: 268–282 (1965).

The effects of maternal morbidity within the 3-month period prior to conception and that following conception, as well as prior pregnancy experience, were examined in relation to pregnancy outcome, especially fetal loss, prematurity, and congenital anomalies. Data were collected on 15 000 American women whose records of medical care during these periods were available. Their infants were followed for 2 years. The classifications of maternal morbidity and congenital anomalies were discussed.

The authors found that: 1 out of 4 pregnancies ended in loss or disability (including minor incapacities); there was a strong relationship between prior pregnancy history and outcome of current pregnancy; and early antepartum bleeding was associated with a high fetal loss rate, as well as with risk of low birth weight, congenital anomalies and neonatal mortality among surviving infants.

SHAPIRO, S. ET AL. Relevance of correlates of infant deaths for significant morbidity at 1 year of age. *American journal of obstetrics and gynecology*, **136**: 363–373 (1980).

To determine whether risk factors for death in the first year of life are also risks for morbidity in surviving infants, data on 390 425 live births, 5084 infant deaths and 4327 surviving 1-year-old children in 8 regions of the USA were examined. Results indicated that factors which presented risks for neonatal death, such as advanced maternal age and maternal history of prior fetal loss, also presented risks for congenital anomalies and/or severe developmental delay. Factors influenced by environmental conditions, such as young maternal age and lower maternal educational attainment, were associated with higher postneonatal mortality rates and significant illnesses among infants of both low and normal birth weight. The choice of parameters for the study was discussed.

SOGBANMU, M. Perinatal mortality and maternal mortality in General Hospital, Ondo, Nigeria; use of high risk pregnancy predictive scoring index. *Nigerian medical journal*, **9**: 123–127 (1979).

Data on perinatal and maternal mortality in 2083 deliveries at General Hospital, Ondo, Nigeria, in 1973 were presented. A scoring system was introduced to identify high-risk patients. Points were assigned for such factors as: sociogeographical information, including residence in a remote area and tribal membership, previous obstetric history, and general medical risk based on clinical examination. On the basis of this system, patients were assigned either to a normal or to a high-risk clinic.

The overall perinatal mortality rate was 52.3 per 1000; intrapartum asphyxia was the most frequent cause. The maternal mortality rate was 7.2 per 1000, caused mainly by anaemia, ruptured uterus, infections, eclampsia, and postpartum haemorrhage. The author noted that certain nonmedical factors, such as failure of the hospital's electricity supply and lack of catering facilities in the hospital, contributed to the high mortality rates. High-risk scores were not compared with perinatal or maternal mortality.

SWENSON, I. & HARPER, P. High risk maternal factors related to fetal wastage in rural Bangladesh. *Journal of biosocial science*, **11**: 465–471 (1979).

Data on pregnancy outcomes collected at the Cholera Research Laboratory in rural Bangladesh from 1966 to 1969 indicated that early fetal wastage and stillbirth among pregnancy orders 1 and 6 or higher were more frequent than among orders 2 and 3. Increased risk was particularly apparent in pregnancies following 2 or more previous fetal deaths.

The authors stated that these results were due to the virtual absence of obstetric care and the high maternal mortality rate in this region, as a result of which only women without reproductive impairment could reach higher parity.

VACCA, A. & BIRD, G. C. Maternal mortality in Papua New Guinea. *Papua New Guinea medical journal*, **20**: 180–186 (1977).

Reports relating to 322 maternal deaths that occurred in Papua New Guinea during the period 1973–1975 were analysed. Of the women concerned, 55% had one or more antepartum risk factors. Causes of death were classified; about 80% were considered preventable within the framework of existing maternal health services. Prevention would depend on the recognition and correct referral of high-risk mothers. The importance of health education and family planning was also stressed.

Summary

Considerable efforts have gone into the creation and improvement of health services, but there are still many areas in the world where access to health care is limited for most of the population. High-quality medical services may be available to prosperous individuals, but universal coverage, at the primary level, is limited by resource constraints such as lack of money and trained manpower. There is thus a need to seek ways of making optimum use of existing resources for the benefit of the majority if the goal of health for all by the year 2000 is to be achieved.

1. The *risk approach* is both a method of measuring the need of individuals and groups for care (thus providing a means of assisting them to determine their priorities) and a tool for the reappraisal and reorganization of health and other services to meet that need. Its aim is to improve care for all, and at the same time to pay special attention to those in greater need. It is thus not fully egalitarian in its approach but shows how to discriminate in favour of the needy in proportion to their need.

2. *Risk factors* are detectable characteristics or circumstances of individuals or groups that are associated with an increased probability ("risk") of having or developing an undesirable condition.

Teenage pregnancy, pregnancy over the age of 40, high parity, too-frequent pregnancies, previous child loss, malnutrition and poor obstetric services are risk factors which increase the chances of a number of undesirable outcomes of pregnancy. For the infant, large families, early weaning, crowding, parental illiteracy and poor sanitation are risk factors for post-neonatal infection and mortality. Certain risk factors are specific to particular outcomes: more often, one risk factor—grand multiparity, for example—increases the likelihood of a number of undesirable outcomes. Most frequently, a number of risk factors combine to endanger further the woman and her infant.

Risk factors may be truly causative, such as hypertension in pregnancy and maternal mortality; on the other hand, they may be merely contributory to the undesired outcome, or they may be predictive only in a statistical sense—for example, illiteracy for perinatal mortality, where the measurable risk factor is a proxy for a number of ill-defined conditions all associated with poverty.

In some situations, culture and custom may act as risk factors by limiting the education or status of women, by prescribing or withholding certain foods during pregnancy or by perpetuating unhygienic practices. In others, the absence or poor quality of health personnel, or the lack of rapid transport to hospital in urgent cases, increases the risks for both mothers and children. Risk factors are thus characteristics not only of individuals and groups, but also of the health and other service sectors and of the social, economic and political environment.

3. The *measurement of risk factors* requires a knowledge of the natural history of complications of labour and pregnancy, of the disorders of infancy and childhood (and of disease generally), as well as a study of the epidemiology of each defined outcome within the local setting. Thus the chain of events can be established and the relevant risk factors for each outcome defined and quantified. It will then be possible to select the risk factors that are most suitable for detection and assessment at different levels of sophistication and to plan the intervention strategy. Some potential factors, such as maternal age, parity and economic status, are easily ascertained by the untrained health worker or by members of the family. Others, such as blood pressure, fetal lie, blood chemistry or water supply quality, require increasing levels of training and resources to measure or detect.

Decisions will have to be made locally as to cut-off points: for instance, should special attention be given to all women who have had 5 children or more, or should it be restricted to those who have had 8 children or more? This will depend on the association between parity and outcome in the community and on the resources available for intervention; likewise, the consequences of "false positives" and "false negatives" (see section 3.5) will need to be taken into account.

The prevalence of risk factors in the community and the ease or feasibility of intervention in each case will decide the priorities. This decision can be facilitated by the computation of the relative risk of undesired outcomes for individuals, groups or environments with defined characteristics and of attributable risk for the community based on the total prevalence and weight of the relevant risk factors (see sections 3.3.2 and 3.3.3).

4. *Intervention strategies based on the risk approach* require, in addition, a careful appraisal of the workings of the health services, plans for their improvement and some estimate of the possibilities for change. This will involve a description of community resources, including health and other social agencies and health and health-related personnel. A *health information system* is an essential part of the risk strategy, providing, at levels consistent with local resources, information on the populations at risk, the services provided, their utilization, and the

results achieved. This knowledge can then be used to extend coverage, to change practices and to modify the referral chain on the basis of the best "match" of need with facility. Such reorganization, with continuous monitoring and feedback, has clear implications for training and supervision and for the organization of the health services generally.

5. The risk approach can be used to improve the health of mothers and children at several levels *both within and outside the health care system*. It is both flexible and resilient, and, as a way of thinking, can be readily adapted to different systems and cultures.

At its most basic, the information derived from examination of risk can be used for health education and for improving personal and family health care. Involvement of the community in the knowledge of individual and group risk factors should lead to an enhanced awareness of health problems and community action programmes.

Within the health care system, more extensive coverage should be followed by better referral practices to increase congruence between needs and skills. Modification of risk factors comes next—by treatment of individuals, by changes in life-style and by improvement of the environment. This will require the adaptation of facilities and skills to meet the different needs both at the local level and at the regional and national levels. Appraisal of regional and national needs for care, based on the distribution of risk, should contribute to the reorganization of the health services and to the revision of plans for health manpower development.

The influence of the health services on the health of the population is limited and the risk approach should clearly indicate the involvement of other sectors in questions of health and disease. Examples are the need for an agricultural policy that will combat malnutrition, a housing policy that will diminish crowding, and a public transport policy that will facilitate access to health services. Thus the risk approach, if taken seriously, has the most important consequences for public policy and can provide the information necessary for intersectoral policy decisions which affect health.

6. The *implementation of the risk approach*, while nominally directed at mothers and children, should have effects on the whole organization of the health and social systems. Success will, however, depend first and foremost on an ability and willingness to reallocate resources and on a health care system that is capable of change and eager for improvement. Professional conservatism and political resistance are but two of the many potential barriers to implementation.

WHO publications may be obtained, direct or through booksellers, from:

ALGERIA	Société Nationale d'Edition et de Diffusion, 3 bd Zirout Youcef, ALGIERS
ARGENTINA	Carlos Hirsch SRL, Florida 165, Galerias Güemes, Escritorio 453/465, BUENOS AIRES
AUSTRALIA	Hunter Publications, 58A Gipps Street, COLLINGWOOD, VIC 3066 — Australian Government Publishing Service *(Mail order sales)*, P.O. Box 84, CANBERRA A.C.T. 2600; *or over the counter from:* Australian Government Publishing Service Bookshops *at:* 70 Alinga Street, CANBERRA CITY A.C.T. 2600; 294 Adelaide Street, BRISBANE, Queensland 4000; 347 Swanston Street, MELBOURNE, VIC 3000; 309 Pitt Street, SYDNEY, N.S.W. 2000; Mt Newman House, 200 St. George's Terrace, PERTH, WA 6000; Industry House, 12 Pirie Street, ADELAIDE, SA 5000; 156–162 Macquarie Street, HOBART, TAS 7000 — R. Hill & Son Ltd., 608 St. Kilda Road, MELBOURNE, VIC 3004; Lawson House, 10–12 Clark Street, CROW'S NEST, NSW 2065
AUSTRIA	Gerold & Co., Graben 31, 1011 VIENNA 1
BANGLADESH	The WHO Programme Coordinator, G.P.O. Box 250, DHAKA 5 — The Association of Voluntary Agencies, P.O. Box 5045, DHAKA 5
BELGIUM	*For books:* Office International de Librairie s.a., avenue Marnix 30, 1050 BRUSSELS. *For periodicals and subscriptions:* Office International des Périodiques, avenue Marnix 30, 1050 BRUSSELS — *Subscriptions to World Health only:* Jean de Lannoy, 202 avenue du Roi, 1060 BRUSSELS
BHUTAN	see India, WHO Regional Office
BOTSWANA	Botsalo Books (Pty) Ltd., P.O. Box 1532, GABORONE
BRAZIL	Biblioteca Regional de Medicina OMS/OPS, Unidade de Venda de Publicações, Caixa Postal 20.381, Vila Clementino, 04023 SÃO PAULO, S.P.
BURMA	see India, WHO Regional Office
CANADA	Canadian Public Health Association, 1335 Carling Avenue, Suite 210, OTTAWA, Ont. K1Z 8N8. *Subscription orders, accompanied by cheque made out to the* Royal Bank of Canada, Ottawa, Account World Health Organization, *may also be sent to the* World Health Organization, PO Box 1800, Postal Station B, OTTAWA, Ont. K1P 5R5
CHINA	China National Publications Import & Export Corporation, P.O. Box 88, BEIJING (PEKING)
CYPRUS	"MAM", P.O. Box 1722, NICOSIA
CZECHO-SLOVAKIA	Artia, Ve Smeckach 30, 111 27 PRAGUE 1
DEMOCRATIC PEOPLE'S REPUBLIC OF KOREA	see India, WHO Regional Office
DENMARK	Munksgaard Export and Subscription Service, Nørre Søgade 35, 1370 COPENHAGEN K (Tel: +45 1 12 85 70)
ECUADOR	Libreria Cientifica S.A., P.O. Box 362, Luque 223, GUAYAQUIL
EGYPT	Osiris Office for Books and Reviews, 50 Kasr El Nil Street, CAIRO
FIJI	The WHO Programme Coordinator, P.O. Box 113, SUVA
FINLAND	Akateeminen Kirjakauppa, Keskuskatu 2, 00101 HELSINKI 10
FRANCE	Librairie Arnette, 2 rue Casimir-Delavigne, 75006 PARIS
GABON	Librairie Universitaire du Gabon, B.P. 3881, LIBREVILLE
GERMAN DEMOCRATIC REPUBLIC	Buchhaus Leipzig, Postfach 140, 701 LEIPZIG
GERMANY, FEDERAL REPUBLIC OF	Govi-Verlag GmbH, Ginnheimerstrasse 20, Postfach 5360, 6236 ESCHBORN — W. E. Saarbach, Postfach 101 610, Follerstrasse 2, 5000 COLOGNE 1 — Alex. Horn, Spiegelgasse 9, Postfach 3340, 6200 WIESBADEN
GHANA	Fides Enterprises, P.O. Box 1628, ACCRA
GREECE	G.C. Eleftheroudakis S.A., Librairie internationale, rue Nikis 4, ATHENS (T. 126)
HAITI	Max Bouchereau, Librairie "A la Caravelle", Boîte postale 111-B, PORT-AU-PRINCE
HONG KONG	Hong Kong Government Information Services, Beaconsfield House, 6th Floor, Queen's Road, Central, VICTORIA
HUNGARY	Kultura, P.O.B. 149, BUDAPEST 62 — Akadémiai Könyvesbolt, Váci utca 22, BUDAPEST V
ICELAND	Snaebjørn Jonsson & Co., P.O. Box 1131, Hafnarstraeti 9, REYKJAVIK
INDIA	WHO Regional Office for South-East Asia, World Health House, Indraprastha Estate, Mahatma Gandhi Road, NEW DELHI 110002 — Oxford Book & Stationery Co., Scindia House, NEW DELHI 110001; 17 Park Street, CALCUTTA 700016 *(Sub-agent)*
INDONESIA	P. T. Kalman Media Pusaka, Pusat Perdagangan Senen, Block 1, 4th Floor, P.O. Box 3433/Jkt, JAKARTA
IRAN (ISLAMIC REPUBLIC OF)	Iran University Press, 85 Park Avenue, P.O. Box 54/551, TEHRAN
IRAQ	Ministry of Information, National House for Publishing, Distributing and Advertising, BAGHDAD
IRELAND	TDC Publishers, 12 North Frederick Street, DUBLIN 1 (Tel: 744835-749677)
ISRAEL	Heiliger & Co., 3 Nathan Strauss Street, JERUSALEM 94227
ITALY	Edizioni Minerva Medica, Corso Bramante 83–85, 10126 TURIN; Via Lamarmora 3, 20100 MILAN
JAPAN	Maruzen Co. Ltd., P.O. Box 5050, TOKYO International, 100–31
JORDAN, THE HASHEMITE KINGDOM OF	Jordan Book Centre Co. Ltd., University Street, P.O. Box 301 (Al-Jubeiha), AMMAN
KUWAIT	The Kuwait Bookshops Co. Ltd., Thunayan Al-Ghanem Bldg, P.O. Box 2942, KUWAIT
LAO PEOPLE'S DEMOCRATIC REPUBLIC	The WHO Programme Coordinator, P.O. Box 343, VIENTIANE
LEBANON	The Levant Distributors Co. S.A.R.L., Box 1181, Makdassi Street, Hanna Bldg, BEIRUT
LUXEMBOURG	Librairie du Centre, 49 bd Royal, LUXEMBOURG
MALAWI	Malawi Book Service, P.O. Box 30044, Chichiti, BLANTYRE 3

A/1/84

WHO publications may be obtained, direct or through booksellers, from:

MALAYSIA	The WHO Programme Coordinator, Room 1004, 10th Floor, Wisma Lim Foo Yong (formerly Fitzpatrick's Building), Jalan Raja Chulan, KUALA LUMPUR 05-10; P.O. Box 2550, KUALA LUMPUR 01-02; Parry's Book Center, K. L. Hilton Hotel, Jln. Treacher, P.O. Box 960, KUALA LUMPUR
MALDIVES	see India, WHO Regional Office
MEXICO	Libreria Internacional, S.A. de C.V., Av. Sonora 206, 06100-MÉXICO, D.F.
MONGOLIA	see India, WHO Regional Office
MOROCCO	Editions La Porte, 281 avenue Mohammed V, RABAT
MOZAMBIQUE	INLD, Caixa Postal 4030, MAPUTO
NEPAL	see India, WHO Regional Office
NETHERLANDS	Medical Books Europe BV, Noorderwal 38, 7241 BL LOCHEM
NEW ZEALAND	Government Printing Office, Publications Section, Mulgrave Street, Private Bag, WELLINGTON 1; Walter Street, WELLINGTON; World Trade Building, Cubacade, Cuba Street, WELLINGTON. *Government Bookshops at:* Hannaford Burton Building, Rutland Street, Private Bag, AUCKLAND; 159 Hereford Street, Private Bag, CHRISTCHURCH; Alexandra Street, P.O. Box 857, HAMILTON; T & G Building, Princes Street, P.O. Box 1104, DUNEDIN — R. Hill & Son Ltd, Ideal House, Cnr Gillies Avenue & Eden Street, Newmarket, AUCKLAND 1
NIGERIA	University Bookshop Nigeria Ltd, University of Ibadan, IBADAN
NORWAY	J. G. Tanum A/S, P.O. Box 1177 Sentrum, OSLO 1
PAKISTAN	Mirza Book Agency, 65 Shahrah-E-Quaid-E-Azam, P.O. Box 729, LAHORE 3; Sasi Limited, Sasi Centre, G.P.O. Box 779, I.I. Chundrigar Road, KARACHI
PAPUA NEW GUINEA	The WHO Programme Coordinator, P.O. Box 646, KONEDOBU
PHILIPPINES	World Health Organization, Regional Office for the Western Pacific, P.O. Box 2932, MANILA — The Modern Book Company Inc., P.O. Box 632, 922 Rizal Avenue, MANILA 2800
POLAND	Składnica Księgarska, ul Mazowiecka 9, 00052 WARSAW *(except periodicals)* — BKWZ Ruch, ul Wronia 23, 00840 WARSAW *(periodicals only)*
PORTUGAL	Livraria Rodrigues, 186 Rua do Ouro, LISBON 2
REPUBLIC OF KOREA	The WHO Programme Coordinator, Central P.O. Box 540, SEOUL
SIERRA LEONE	Njala University College Bookshop (University of Sierra Leone), Private Mail Bag, FREETOWN
SINGAPORE	The WHO Programme Coordinator, 144 Moulmein Road, SINGAPORE 1130; Newton P.O. Box 31, SINGAPORE 9122 — Select Books (Pte) Ltd, 215 Tanglin Shopping Centre, 2/F, 19 Tanglin Road, SINGAPORE 10
SOUTH AFRICA	Van Schaik's Bookstore (Pty) Ltd, P.O. Box 724, 268 Church Street, PRETORIA 0001
SPAIN	Comercial Atheneum S.A., Consejo de Ciento 130-136, BARCELONA 15; General Moscardó 29, MADRID 20 — Libreria Diaz de Santos, Lagasca 95 y Maldonado 6, MADRID 6; Balmes 417 y 419, BARCELONA 22
SRI LANKA	see India, WHO Regional Office
SWEDEN	*For books:* Aktiebolaget C.E. Fritzes Kungl. Hovbokhandel, Regeringsgatan 12, 103 27 STOCKHOLM. *For periodicals:* Wennergren-Williams AB, Box 30004, 104 25 STOCKHOLM
SWITZERLAND	Medizinischer Verlag Hans Huber, Länggass Strasse 76, 3012 BERNE 9
THAILAND	see India, WHO Regional Office
TUNISIA	Société Tunisienne de Diffusion, 5 avenue de Carthage, TUNIS
TURKEY	Haset Kitapevi, 469 Istiklal Caddesi, Beyoglu, ISTANBUL
UNITED KINGDOM	H.M. Stationery Office: 49 High Holborn, LONDON WC1V 6HB; 13a Castle Street, EDINBURGH EH2 3AR; 80 Chichester Street, BELFAST BT1 4JY; Brazennose Street, MANCHESTER M60 8AS; 258 Broad Street, BIRMINGHAM B1 2HE; Southey House, Wine Street, BRISTOL BS1 2BQ. *All mail orders should be sent to:* HMSO Publications Centre, 51 Nine Elms Lane, LONDON SW8 5DR
UNITED STATES OF AMERICA	*Single and bulk copies of individual publications (not subscriptions):* WHO Publications Centre USA, 49 Sheridan Avenue, ALBANY, NY 12210. *Subscriptions: Subscription orders, accompanied by check made out to* the Chemical Bank, New York, Account World Health Organization, *should be sent to the* World Health Organization, PO Box 5284, Church Street Station, NEW YORK, NY 10249; *Correspondence concerning subscriptions should be addressed to the* World Health Organization, Distribution and Sales, 1211 GENEVA 27, Switzerland. *Publications are also available from the* United Nations Bookshop, NEW YORK, NY 10017 *(retail only)*
URUGUAY	Libreria Agropecuaria S. R. L., Casilla de Correo 1755, Alzaibar 1328, MONTEVIDEO
USSR	*For readers in the USSR requiring Russian editions:* Komsomolskij prospekt 18, Medicinskaja Kniga, Moscow — *For readers outside the USSR requiring Russian editions:* Kuzneckij most 18, Meždunarodnaja Kniga, Moscow G-200
VENEZUELA	Libreria del Este, Apartado 60.337, CARACAS 106 — Libreria Médica Paris, Apartado 60.681, CARACAS 106
YUGOSLAVIA	Jugoslovenska Knjiga, Terazije 27/II, 11000 BELGRADE
ZAIRE	Librairie universitaire, avenue de la Paix N° 167, B.P. 1682, KINSHASA I

Special terms for developing countries are obtainable on application to the WHO Programme Coordinators or WHO Regional Offices listed above or to the World Health Organization, Distribution and Sales Service, 1211 Geneva 27, Switzerland. Orders from countries where sales agents have not yet been appointed may also be sent to the Geneva address, but must be paid for in pounds sterling, US dollars, or Swiss francs.

Price: Sw. fr. 11.—   Prices are subject to change without notice.